THE NATURE'S FARMACY

━◄• CHINONSO ANYAEHIE •►━

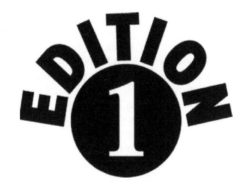

EDITION 1

ISBN: 978-0-692-71204-7
Copyright © 2016 The Nature's Farmacy

Disclaimer

Table of Contents

Dedication 25

Acknowledgements 26

Foreword 28

Introduction 30

Chaptet 1: 50 Marvellous Miracles of Baking Soda   **34**

Fights Acne and Pimples: 36

Teeth Whitener: 36

Treats Sunburn: 37

Improves Skin Complexion: 37

Ulcer Pain: 37

Treats Body Odour: 38

Removes Dandruff: 38

Treats Stained or Yellow Nails: 39

Constipation: 39

Yeast Infection: 40

Upset Stomach: 40

Diaper Rash: 41

Insect Bites and Poison Ivy: 41

Heartburn, Indigestion, and Ulcer Pain: 41

Foot Soak and Exfoliator 42

Relaxing Soak: 42

Enhanced Sports Performance: 42

Splinter Remover: 42

Hand Cleanser: 43

Remove Blackheads: 43

Sweeten Your Tomatoes: 43

Canker Sore: 44

Great Scrub: 44

Pamper Your Feet: 44

Freshen Sponges: 45

Deodorize Garbage Disposals: 45

Get rid of Toilet Odour: 45

Carpet Deodorizer: 45

Dry Shampoo: 45

Volumizing Shampoo: 45
Cleaning Agent: 46
Facial Scrub: 46
Nail Cleaner: 46
Smelly Shoes: 46
Remove Chlorine from Hair: 46
Pedicure: 46
Modelling Clay: 47
Natural Oven Cleaning: 47
Soften Fabric: 47
Silver Polish: 47
Clean Kitchen Utensils: 47
Air freshener: 47
Neutralize Gassy Beans: 48
Produce Wash: 48
Keep Ants Out: 48
Erase Crayon, Pencil, Ink, and Furniture
Scuffs from Painted Surfaces: 48
Deodorize Garbage Cans: 48
Boiling Chicken: 48
Keep Flowers Fresher Longer: 49

Chaptet 2: Amazing Benefits of Enemas   **50**

The Amazing Health Benefits of Coffee Enemas: 51
Epsom Salt Enema: 53
Lemon Juice Enema 54
Salt Water Enema 56
Acidophilus Enema 57

Chaptet 3: Sure-fire Ways to Lose Weight in Ten Days   **58**

Cinnamon: 59
Honey and Cinnamon: 60
Lemon Juice: 60
Water Therapy: 61
Honey & Ginger Remedy: 61
Lemon, Honey, Pepper Remedy: 62
Hot Pepper: 62
Almonds: 63
Apple Cider Vinegar and Water 63
Lemon Juice and Hot Water 64

Dandelion Remedy: 64
Cabbage: 65
Hot Water Remedy: 65
Cucumber Remedy: 66
Green Tea: 66
Garlic and Lemon Remedy 67
Cranberry Juice: 67
Coconut Oil 68
Omega-3 Fatty Acids: 68
Juice Fast: 69
Herbal Cleanse: 69
Deciding What Foods to Eat: 70
Diet Plan/Guidelines: 70

Chaptet 4: **Marvellous Miracles of Honey**   77

The Honey and Cinnamon Cure 78

Chaptet 5: **Must Have Natural Remedies for Any First Aid Kit**   84

Natural First Aid Remedies 85
Tea Tree Oil: 85
Lavender Essential Oil: 86
Clove Oil 87
Aloe Vera Gel 87
Witch Hazel 88
Bach Rescue Remedy 89
Arnica Oil 89
Calendula Cream: 90
Sea Buckthorn Oil 91
Cayenne 92
Ginger 92
Goldenseal 93
Oil of Oregano 93
Neem 94
Licorice tea: 95
Probiotic for Diarrhea: 95
Vitamin D for Flu: 96
Hydrogen Peroxide for Colds and Flu: 96
Ginger for Nausea: 96
Pure Water for Hiccups: 96

Chaptet 6: **Marvellous Miracles of Apple Cider Vinegar**   97

Remove Dandruff 98
Soothe A Sore Throat 98
Diabetes 98
Heart Health 99
Skin Irritation 99
Warts 99
Energy Boost 99
Repel Fleas On Your Pets 99
Reduce Heartburn 100
Balance Your Digestive System 100
Sinus Congestion 100
Helps Get Rid of Candida 100
Clear Up Your Skin 101
Oral Health 101
Deodorant 101
For Hair 101
Asthma 101
Arthritis 102
Athlete's Foot 102
Nose Bleeding 102
Blood Pressure 102
Bone Health 102
Bruises 103
Burns 103
Colds 103
Constipation 103
Diarrhea 103
Ear Infections 104
Eczema 104
Menstrual Problems 104
Leg Cramp 104
Morning Sickness 104
Sore Muscles 104
Fabric Softener 105
Clean Your Washing Machine 105
Hiccups 105
Insect Bites and Stings 105
Boil Eggs 105
Ulcers 105

Urinary Tract Infections 106

Varicose Veins 106

Shingles 106

Corn and Callus Treatment 106

Flatulence 106

Night Sweats and Hot Flashes 106

Clean Barbecue Grill 107

Yeast Infection 107

Sinus 107

Weight Loss 107

Chaptet 7: **Marvellous Miracles of Aloe Vera**   **108**

Aloe Vera for Facial Scrub 110

Treat Burns 110

Treat Scalds 110

Soothe Insect Bites, Stings and Itching 110

Prevent Permanent Tissue Damage From Frostbite With Aloe 111

Aloe for Rashes and Allergic Reactions 111

Help Heal Herpes Outbreaks 111

Fight Athlete's Foot 111

Prevent Pimples and Treat Acne 112

Soothe Psoriasis with Aloe Vera 112

Prevent Scarring and Stretch Marks 113

Help Get Rid of Rosacea 113

Shrink Warts 113

Reduce Wrinkles and Rejuvenate with Aloe 113

Help Eliminate Eczema 114

Encourage Hair Growth: Clean Out Your Hair Pores with Aloe 114

Aloe For Your Exfoliating Experiments 114

Soothing Aloe Vera and Baking Soda Scrub 115

Homemade Olive Oil, Aloe, and Sugar Scrub 115

Reduce Hair Dandruff 115

Replace Aloe with Conditioner for Silkier, Smoother hair 115

Makeup Remover 115

Treat Minor Vaginal Irritations 116

Drink Aloe Vera Juice to Relieve Gastrointestinal Disorders Like Indigestion 116

For Rheumatoid Arthritis Pain 116

Alleviate Asthma 116

Drink to Lower Blood Sugar Levels—Especially for Diabetics. 117

Aloe Vera For Bad Breath 117

Aloe As A Sore Throat Remedy 117

Aloe Vera for Receding Gums 117

Aloe for Acid Reflux Relief 118

A Natural Treatment For Conjunctivitis 118

Get Rid of Contusion 118

Aloe Vera For Constipation 118

Aloe Vera For Heat Rash 119

Aloe For A Healthier Heart 119

Chaptet 8: **Amazing Uses of Hydrogen Peroxide**   120

Get rid of acne and boils 121

Replace Chlorine 121

Cure Canker Sores 121

Bad Breath 121

Fight Food Fungus 121

Treat Cold / Flu 121

Get Rid of Ear infections and Clear Out Ear Wax 122

Sinus Infections 122

Tackle Toothache 122

Take A Detoxifying Bath 122

Yeast Infections 122

Deodorant 123

Clean Your Contact Lenses 123

Tile and Grout Scrub 123

Whiten Your Nails 123

Laundry Bleach 123

Fruit and Veggie Sanitizer 123

Odor Eliminator 124

Lighten Your Hair 124

Disinfect Your Toothbrushes 124

Soften Calluses and Corns 124

Disinfect Small Wounds 124

Help Heal Boils 124

Disinfect Your Countertops 124

Clean Your Mirrors 124

Wash Out Your Toilet Bowl 125

Remove Tub Scum 125

To Clean Grout / Tiles 125

Kill Mold 125

Canine Emetic 125

Bloodstain Remover 126

Keep Salad Fresh 126

Vegetable Soak 126

Get Rid of Stubborn Caked On Foods 126

Chaptet 9: **Marvellous Miracles of Coconut Oil**   127

Weight Loss 128

Prevent Stretch Marks 128

Cold Sores 128

Energy 128

Yeast Infections 128

Moisturize Your Skin 128

Conditioner 129

Reduce Risk (or effect) of Alzheimer's 129

Make Homemade Soap 129

Shaving "Cream" 129

Deodorant 130

Lip Balm 131

Dog Diet 131

Coffee Creamer 132

Antibacterial 132

Wood Polish 132

Heart Disease 133

Lower Cholesterol 133

Soothe Fly Bites 134

Acne Remedy 134

Oil/Butter Replacement 134

Exfoliating Body Scrub 134

Makeup Remover 135

Massage Oil 135

Nail and Cuticle Treatment 136

Diaper Cream 136

Nipple Cream 136

Fight Inflammation 136

Leather Polish 137

Remove Chewing Gum 137

Get Rid of Soap Scum 137

Season Cast Iron Pans 137

Bath Oil 138

HIV – AIDS 138

Rash Soother 139

Reduce Dandruff 139

Remove Rust 139

Prevent Split Ends 139

Sore throat 139

Treat Athletes Foot 140

Popcorn Topping 140

Used As Toothpaste 140

Sunscreen 141

Wound Care 141

Insect Repellent 141

Bee Sting Soother 141

Frizz Fighter 141

Metal Polish 141

Moisten Chapped Nose 141

Coconut Oil Pulling 142

Increase Milk Flow 142

Circumcision Healing 142

Eyelash Enhancement 142

Preserve Eggs 143

Grease Baking Pans 143

Lubricate Kitchen Appliances 143

Prevent Morning Sickness 143

Cheekbone Highlighter 143

Shape Your Beard / Moustache 143

Detail Your Car 143

Constipation Relief. 144

Prevent Perineum Tears 144

Cream Foundation Base 144

Wrinkle Buster 144

Mascara Brush Cleaner 144

Visibly Brighter Skin 144

Foot Exfoliator 144

Use at Bath Time 144

Easy to Clean Baby Bottom 145

Goodbye Baby Lotion 145

Target Eczema and Psoriasis 145

Treat Baby Thrush 145

Help Your Baby Develop 145

Help Provide Teething Relief in Babies 145

Natural Baby Massage Oil 145
Constipation Relief in Babies 146
Lip Exfoliator 146
Maintain Lawn Mower Blades 146
Hay Fever 146
Prevent Lice 146
Aromatherapy 146
Dry Nostrils 146
Fade Age/Sun Spots 147
Bags-Be-Gone 147
Soften Dry Elbows 147
Give Your Dog a Healthy Shine 147
Heal Wounds 147
Soothe a Dry Canine Nose 147
Ease Arthritis Pain 147
Flaky Scalp Treatment: 148
Reduce Fine Lines: 148
Fight Ringworm: 148
Ease Osteoporosis: 148
Help Heal a Bruise 149
Food Poisoning Relief 149
Tattoo Moisturizer/Healer 149
Dust Repellent 149
Cutting Board Conditioner 149
 Go-To Carrier/Base Oil 149
DIY Vapor Rub 150
On Toast 150
Small Motor Lubricant 150
Cracked Paw Pads 150
Give Plants a Shine 150
Get Rid of Cradle Cap 150
Improve blood circulation 150
Ink Cleaner 151
Breath Freshener 151
Personal Lubricant 151
Detangler 151
Natural face mask 151
Treat enlarged prostate 151
Urinary tract infection (UTI) 152
Protozoal infections 152

Pre-workout supplement 152
Seizure reduction 152

Chaptet 10: **Water Therapy and Infused Water**   **153**

Lemon Infused Water: 155
Apple Cinnamon Water Recipe: 156
Lemon Lime Infuse Water 157
Lemon Cucumber Water: 158

Chaptet 11: **Marvellous Miracles of Epson Salt**   **159**

Foot soak / pedicure 160
Soak sprains and bruises 161
End constipation 161
Hangover cure 161
Face cleaner 161
Skin exfoliator 161
Remove excess oil from hair 162
Remove hairspray 162
Hair volumizer: 162
Eye wash 162
Relieve minor irritation 162
Relieve gout 162
Remove blackheads 163
Make grass greener 163
Insecticide spray 163
Beautiful roses 163
Bigger, better, and more produce 163
Get rid of raccoons 164
Clean bathroom tiles 164
Remove burnt foot from pot and pans 164
Regenerate your car battery 164
Help kids sleep better 164
Get rid of slugs 164
Sore muscles and splinters 165

Chaptet 12: **Home Remedies for Constipation**   **166**

Take castor oil. 167
Baking soda 167
Lemon 168

Aloe Vera 168

Fennel Tea 168

Figs 169

Honey 169

Flaxseed 170

Grapes 170

Fiber 170

Prunes 171

Molasses 171

Avoid cheese and dairy products. 172

Chaptet 13: **Home Remedies for Menstrual Cramp**   **173**

Ginger: 174

Cinnamon: 174

Chamomile Tea: 175

Parsley: 175

Peppermint: 175

Basil: 176

Heat or Hot Compress: 176

Exercise: 176

Prevention Tips 176

Chaptet 14: **Basic Beauty Routine**   **178**

Cleansing: 179

Yogurt, Oatmeal, and Cucumber: 180

Un-Boiled Milk: 180

Avocado: 180

Tomato, Milk, and Lemon Juice: 180

Toning: 181

Moisturizing: 181

Additional Facial Skin Care Tips: 181

Chaptet 15: **Home Remedies For Snoring**   **183**

Lifestyle Remedies for Snoring 184

Use a Tennis Ball 185

Use a Backpack 185

Elevate Your Head 186

Gargle with Peppermint 186

Inhaling steam 186

Nettle Leaf Tea Remedy for Snoring 187

Garlic Remedies for snoring 187

Mint Tea 187

Chaptet 16: Amazing uses of lemon for beauty   189

Blackhead: 190

Elbow and knee bleacher: 190

Canker sore treatment: 190

Clarifying moisturizer: 190

Cleansing wipes: 190

Get rid of wrinkles: 190

Teeth whitener: 191

Lighten / brighten Your Skin: 191

Lips exfoliator: 191

Hair Lightener: 191

Tone up your Skin: 191

Nail strengthener: 191

Shine Eliminator: 192

Moisturize Your Skin: 192

When using lemon I want you to take note of these few pointers. 192

Chaptet 17: Home Remedies for Dandruff   193

Lemon for Dandruff 194

Baking Soda for Dandruff 194

Aloe Vera for Dandruff 195

Ginger for dandruff 196

Apple Cider Vinegar and Dandruff 197

Chaptet 18: Alternative Treatment for Canker Sore   198

Baking Soda 199

Onion 199

Coriander 200

Hydrogen Peroxide 200

Sea Salt & Honey Rub 200

Aloe Vera 201

Coconut Oil 201

Cayenne Pepper 202

Sage Tea Rinse 202

Honey 202

Tea Tree 203

Chamomile Tea Bag 203

Dehydrate your canker sore with Milk of Magnesia. 204

Chaptet 19: **Get Rid of Dark Circles Naturally**   **205**

Cucumber: 206

Rose Water: 206

Almond Oil: 206

Tomato: 207

Raw Potato: 207

Turmeric: 207

Lemon Juice: 207

Mint Leaves: 208

Apple: 208

Chamomile Tea Bags: 208

Chaptet 20: **Homemade honey facial masks**   **210**

Avocado Honey Mask for Dry Skin 210

Tightening Egg White Mask 211

Anti-Aging Flaxseed + Honey Mask 211

Anti-Acne Lemon Yogurt + Honey Mask 211

Cinnamon Honey Mask 212

Chaptet 21: **Banana Facial Mask**   **213**

Banana, Honey, and Lemon Juice Face Mask 214

Acne-Fighting Banana Face Mask 214

Wrinkle Removing Banana Face Mask 215

Moisture Locking Banana Mask: 215

Chaptet 22: **13 Herbal Remedies for Glowing Skin**   **217**

Grapes: 218

Cucumber juice, glycerine and rose water: 218

Sandalwood, turmeric, and milk: 218

Fresh milk, salt, and lime juice: 218

Tomato and lemon juice: 218

Turmeric powder, wheat flour, and sesame oil: 218

 Cabbage juice and honey: 218

Carrot juice: 218

Honey and cinnamon powder 219
Groundnut oil and lime juice: 219
Aloe Vera juice: 219
Ghee and glycerine: 219
Apricots and yogurt: 219

Chaptet 23: **The Most Effective Remedies for hair Growth**   **220**

Onion juice: 221
Potato Juice 221
Eggs White, Olive Oil, and Honey 222
Rinse Hair with Apple Cider Vinegar 222
Use Fenugreek 222
Ayurvedic Herbs – Indian Gooseberry 223

Chaptet 24: **Cucumber mask for a fresh and smooth skin**   **224**

Cucumber Mask #1 225
Cucumber Mask #2 225
Cucumber Mask #3 226
Cucumber Mask #4 226
Cucumber Mask #5 227
Cucumber Mask #6 227
Natural Beauty tips when using Cucumber Face Masks 228

Chaptet 25: **Effective Ways to tighten Loose Vagina**   **229**

Pueraria Mirifica 231
Oak Gall 231
Kegel Exercise 232
Vaginal Cone 232
Ben-wa balls 232
Leg Raise 233

Chaptet 26: **Ways to enlarge your breast naturally**   **234**

Fenugreek 235
Breast Massage 236
Skin Brushing or Fat Transfer Massage. 237
Exercise 237
Amino Acids 237
Vitamins 237

Herbs 238

Pueraria Mirifica 238

Saw palmetto 238

Dong quai 238

Wild yam 239

Damiana 239

Fennel Seeds 239

Red Clover: 239

Chaptet 27: **Treat Hair loss with these Herbal Remedies**   240

Fenugreek seed for Balding 241

Henna for Balding 241

Camphor oil for Balding 241

Lemon Seeds and Peppercorns for Balding 242

Onion for Balding 242

Honey and Onion for Balding 242

Aloe Vera for Hairloss 242

Saw Palmetto for Balding 243

Castor Oil for Balding 243

Hibiscus for Balding 244

Olive Oil for Baldness 244

Chaptet 28: **Effective Home Remedies for Wrinkles**   246

Diet Remedies for Wrinkles: 247

Drink plenty of Water 247

Have foods with wrinkle fighting elements 247

Lifestyle Remedies for Wrinkles 248

Sleep sufficient and sleep right: 248

Don't Stress: 248

 Avoid smoking, alcohol and caffeine 249

Protect and preserve yourself from wrinkle forming sources 249

Protect skin from harmful sun-rays 249

Use cosmetics with care 249

Powerful home Remedies for Wrinkles 250

Avocado Mask 250

Papaya-Banana Mask 250

Egg White Wonder 251

Honey 251

Olive Oil- Pineapple Mask 252

Curd and Turmeric Face Mask For Wrinkles 252

Coconut Oil 252

Turmeric- Sugarcane Mask 252

Vitamin E Mask 253

Papaya, Banana, & Honey 253

Chaptet 29: **Papaya for youthful skin**   256

Papaya for Acne 258

Papaya, Cucumber Banana Facial Mask 258

Papaya and Egg White Face Mask 259

Papaya and Milk cream 259

Wrinkles: 260

Lightens Unwanted Facial Hair 260

Heals Cracked Heels 261

Controls Dandruff 261

Chaptet 30: **Apple cider vinegar for Eczema**   262

Why is vinegar so potent in the treatment of eczema? 263

How to use Apple Cider Vinegar for Eczema 263

ACV Diluted in Water 263

Apple Cider Vinegar Bath 264

Taking ACV Orally 264

Apple Cider Vinegar and Baking Soda 264

Apple Cider Vinegar and Honey 265

Chaptet 31: **Techniques to Prevent Premature Ejaculation**   267

Types of Premature Ejaculation 268

Techniques to Delay Ejaculation
Self-Stimulation: 268

Scrotal Pull: 268

Think Nonsexual Thoughts: 268

External Prostate Spot: 269

Pc (Pubococcygeous) Muscle Contraction: 269

The Squeeze Technique: 269

Breathing: 269

Focus on Foreplay: 269

Take It Slow: 270

Chaptet 32: **Effective Remedies for Kidney Stones**   271

Some Symptoms Includes: 272

Recommendations 272

Watermelon: 273

Aloe Vera: 273

Apple Cider Vinegar: 273

Lemon Juice and Olive Oil: 273

Pomegranate 274

Nettle Tea 274

Nettle Leaf 274

How to Make a Nettle Infusion 275

Basil 275

Wheatgrass 275

Celery 276

Tomatoes 276

Kidney Beans 276

Bran Flakes 276

Chaptet 33: **Home Remedies for Removing Gallstones**   278

Home Remedies for Removing Gallstones 279

The Gallbladder Cleanse: 279

Drinking Oil 280

Reactions to Cleanse 280

The Fourth Day (Passing the Stone) 280

Beetroot, Cucumber and Carrot Juice for Gallstones ... 281

Apple Juice and Apple Cider Vinegar for Gallstones 281

Pear Juice 282

Milk Thistle for Gallstones 282

Dandelion for Gallstones 283

Lemon Juice for Gallstone 283

Psyllium: 283

Peppermint for Gallstones 284

Diet Tips for Gallstones 284

Chaptet 34: **Alternative Treatment for Yeast Infection**   286

Yogurt Remedy for Yeast 287

Garlic Treatment 287

Grapefruit Seed Extract for Yeast Infection 288

Coconut Oil for Yeast Infection 288

How to Use Coconut Oil for Yeast Infection (Topical Application) 289

Essential Oils for Yeast Infection 290

Vinegar for Yeast Infection 290

Chaptet 35: **Untold Psoriasis Treatment, Revealed!** 292

Slippery ELM 293

American Yellow Saffron Herbal Tea. 293

Psoriatrax 293

Fish Oil 294

Tunn off the Nightshade: 294

Foods to avoid 295

Tea Tree Oil 295

Aloe Vera 296

Capsaicin 296

Oat Bath 297

Vinegar Dip 297

Turmeric: 298

Included in your daily diet 298

Castor Oil 298

Chaptet 36: **Effective cures for Shingles** 299

Effective Home Remedies for Shingles Honey for Shingles 300

Baking Soda or Cornstarch 300

Apple Cider Vinegar: 301

Aloe Vera and Cayenne Pepper 301

Turmeric 301

Use a Wet Compress. 302

Try Epsom Salt 302

Use Calamine Lotion 302

Garlic 303

Oatmeal 303

Chaptet 37: **Amazing uses of Turmeric as First Aid** 305

Turmeric for Skin Problems: 306

Depression: 306

Turmeric for diabetes 307

Turmeric for Asthma 308

Rheumatoid Arthritis 308

Cancer 309

Brain Health and Memory 309

Stomach Disorders: 309
Turmeric for Urinary 310
Turmeric for teeth whitening 310
Turmeric for scalp 310
Liver Diseases 311
Skin and Aging 311

Chaptet 38: An Abscessed Tooth? Here are the remedies   312

Water and Salt Rinse 313
Oil Pulling 313
Garlic 314
Wet Black Tea Bag 314
Hydrogen Peroxide 314
Apple Cider Vinegar 315
Turmeric 315
Oregano Oil 316
Peppermint Oil 316
Potato 316
Chamomile 317
Echinacea 317
Additional Tips 317

Chaptet 39: Effective treatment for Asthma   319

Magnesium Supplement 320
Boswellia 320
Mullein Oil 320
Mustard Oil 320
Ginger 320
Garlic 321
Nettle Tea 321
Figs 321
Honey 322
Onions 322
Rosemary Tea. 322
Lemon 322
Safflower Seeds 322
Licorice 323
Steam Inhalation 323

Chaptet 40:   **Banish Acne with these simple remedies**   **324**

Baking Soda 325
Tea Tree 325
Lemon 326
Honey 326
Toothpaste 327
Oatmeal 327
loe Vera 328
Turmeric 328
Apple Cider Vinegar 328
Raw Tomatoes 329
Egg White 329
Papaya for a pimple prone 330
Orange Peels 330
Potato Acne Remedy 330
Fenugreek 331
Indian lilac 331
Aspirin Paste 331
Make a sea salt mixture. 332
Fuller's Earth 332

Chaptet 41:   **Efficient Remedies to Remove Stretch Marks**   **333**

Potato for Stretch Marks: 334
Lemon Juice 334
Egg Whites 335
Aloe Vera 335
Castor Oil 335
Apricot Mask 336
Alfalfa Leaves 336
Coco-Shea Butter 336
Sugar 337
Olive Oil 337
Water 337

Chaptet 42:   **Removing blackhead with home remedies.**   **338**

The Honey Remedy 339
Honey and Milk Pore Strips 339
Egg White Mask 339
Baking Soda 340

Sugar Scrub: 341

Lemon 341

Steam It Out 342

Chaptet 43: **Amazing treatment for Uterine Fibroid**   **343**

Green Tea 344

Flaxseed: 345

Vitex (Vitex Agnus-Castus) 345

Dandelion Root (Taraxacum Officinale) 345

Milk thistle (Silybum Marianum) 345

Nettle (Urtica Dioica) 346

Yellow Dock (Rumex Crispus) 346

Red Raspberry 346

Herbal Tea (Red Clover) 346

Herbal Bath 347

Essential Oil Supplements 347

Avoid High estrogen foods: 347

Decrease the intake of white food: 347

Consume more fiber and soy: 348

Acupuncture: 348

Chinese Medicine: 348

Chaptet 44: **Colon Cleansing Made Easy**   **349**

3 Days Apple Juice Fast 350

Sea Salt 350

Triphala (Ayurvedic Herbal Remedy for Colon Cleansing) 351

Water 351

Fruits and Vegetables high in fiber- for everyday colon cleansing 352

Lemon Juice 352

Chaptet 45: **Reversing Diabetes**   **353**

Fenugreek Remedies for Diabetes 354

Bilberry Extract 355

Bitter Gourd 355

Cinnamon Remedies for Diabetes 356

Aloe Vera Remedy for Diabetes 357

Lady Finger for Diabetes 357

Papaya Leaf Remedies for Diabetes 357

Mango Leaves Remedies for Diabetes 358

How to use Mango Leaves for Diabetes 358
Get Physical 358
Change your Diet 359

Index 360
Bibliography 363

Dedication

I have this blank page to express my undying loving for just a few people close to my heart. The words shown on this page is more than anything money can buy. I went through hell and high water to write this book, and if you are reading this, then my perseverance paid off. Now I write their names in the sands of time. I pray that after our time here on earth, we all meet again in Heaven. They are no other people than my family. Kosisochi Anyaehie (Sister), Lotachi Anyaehie (Sister), Chibuzo Anyaehie (Sister), Odilia Anyaehie (Mom) Emmanuel Anyaehie (Dad), Benedict Oji (Aunty)

Acknowledgements

After three years of wanting to write this book, I have finally gotten the nerve to put down something. After series of severe rock bottom situations, depression, and searching for my purpose here on earth, I have chosen to embark on this journey as part of my life work. This wouldn't have been possible without a set of individuals who assisted me in several ways – by their support and goodwill. When I felt like all hope was lost, they rekindled the fire in me and urged me to keep pushing on.

I can confidently say that this book wouldn't have been possible if they hadn't been a part of my life. In my next life, I pray that I meet people like them. They have not only shown me support, but have also become friends and like family to me. I have met and dealt with a lot of bad people in the past who have robbed me of my joy and made me less of a believer in humanity, but meeting these people has proven to me that there is still love out there on earth. If I had gold and silver, I would give to them. If there is any way to be a real life Super Man, I will become one for them. I hate fair-weather friends; people who are just in your life for what they can get from you, but these individuals have distinguished themselves and shown me that they have my best interests at heart. Even at my very worst, they understood me. Even when I neglected them, they prayed for me, and whenever I retraced my steps, they accepted me. I pray for God's blessings on them. At the top of the list is my very own mother, Mrs. Odilia Anyaehie Listing all she has done for me would be like starting a new book, so I had better not say much! Aunty Benedict Oji, my mother's sister, is an angel living amongst men. On several occasions, I had gone astray, but this woman kept putting me in line with her prayers and support. My sisters Kosiso, Lotachi, Chibuzo are perfect sisters given to me by God; I couldn't ask for more. Their impact and support in my life have led me this far.

I will forever be grateful to my dad, Mr. Emmanuel Anyaehie, for all he has taught me. I am also indebted to my grandmother. If not for her wisdom and teachings, this book wouldn't have been possible.

Also on the list is Jackie Woodside, the author of Calming the Chaos. I have never met an individual with such a beautiful soul before. We are worlds apart geographically and from different races but she believed in me, saw greatness in me, and her encouraging words will always remain in my heart. Whenever I feel like giving up, I remember the promises I made to her; and that keeps me going.

To my other friends Tito Amuchenwa, Jed Mark Serilla, Mr and Mrs Awoba-sivwe, and Aitty Moore: Those constant calls to see that this book was published propelled me to take action. ¬What else can I say, but that I appreciate you all.

Foreword

I had the pleasure of meeting Chinonso Anyaehie on social media and was immediately captured with the depth and breadth of his knowledge about health and wellness. Not only was I impressed with who he is as an author and wellness professional, but I was also more inspired by his deep-seated passion for wellbeing. He understands that everything is energy and that we need to put pure, healthy energies in our bodies when they are compromised in any way to aid healing. He has put together an incredible "encyclopedia" of nature's remedies here in Nature's Farmacy.

Prepare to enter the fascinating world of natural remedies. Nature's Farmacy offers readers an array of approaches for numerous health and wellness issues, challenges, and ailments. There is an intuitive knowing that comes from reading this book that nature finds a way to heal it's own ailments and cure its illnesses.

From bad breath to body odor, insect bites to skin problems and even natural remedies for breast enlargement, you will find natural solutions and resources for all kinds of common health concerns. Your spouse's snoring keeping you up at night? Not a problem when you know the natural solutions for addressing it. Irritable bowel problems, constipation and other ailments of the gut are addressed in detail. Every imaginable ailment has a natural solution, and you will find what you need in this incredibly detailed summary called Nature's Farmacy.

Nature's Farmacy details the numerous benefits of everyday products that you likely already have in your kitchen. You probably did not know that there are fifty different ways that Apple Cider Vinegar can be used to improve health and wellbeing or that Epsom Salts offers 25 different benefits! These are just a small sampling of the depth of Nature's Farmacy information waiting for you to discover and enjoy.

Chinonso Anyaehie is truly an expert. Not only is he an expert in his knowledge base, but he is one who walks this talk. Living in Nigeria where political and social conditions can sometimes be harsh and unpredictable, he maintains an incredible sense of wellness, optimism, and complete wellness despite the challenges of his native land.

No matter what health challenge you are facing, Nature's Farmacy has a solution. The pharmaceutical industry would have us believe that we need chemicals to resolve our bodies ailments. Not so! The wisdom of Nature's Farmacy brings forth the truth that what our bodies need is already present in nature itself. We simply need to educate ourselves as to what to use, in what combinations, to address which ailments we face.

Jackie Woodside
Author of Calming the Chaos: A Soulful Guide to Managing your Energy Rather than Your Time and Time for a Change: Essential Skills for Managing the Inevitable

Introduction

This book is nothing but an accumulation of my personal experience with home remedies and everything that has happened to me up until now as I have experimented with these remedies. Within the pages of this book are timeless nuggets of wisdom and knowledge, given to me by my grandparents.

After I left my parents and grandparents to journey far away to the big city in search of greener pastures, I was exposed to a whole new world, where most people lived their lives on autopilot without taking the necessary time to live in the present and take care of their health. Life in the big city is something I pray that I would be able to escape from one day. Trust me. I don't think I have enough strength to compete for any position or fight for anything with anyone. I have come to a point in my life where I need nothing but absolute peace of mind and joy. I wish to live a life free from resentment, hate, and regrets. I spent seven years of my life climbing the corporate ladder, and suddenly when I thought I was making headway, I got crushed so badly that I landed below where I started from. Now, I have another opportunity to begin again and this time, I'm doing things differently and choosing a whole new path to life. In this book, I have shared a few home remedies I have personally tried out and have also recommended to few friends in the past few years. Those who have tried my solutions, came back with positive testimonials. I have used my personal stories to illustrate how these remedies work, so it would be easier for you to understand. I'm currently working on more remedies which I will include in the subsequent editions of this book.

Most of the remedies in this book are gotten from my grandmother's healing journal. My grandmother is a well-known herbalist and spiritual teacher and has cured hundreds of people with her natural and holistic approach. I was my grandmother's greatest cheerleader. It was a great privilege working with a known healer. I was more or less her personal assistant, and if you needed her assistance, you had to go through me. I ran errands and cultivated most of the herbs she used for her work. I guessed that my love for natural healing started at a very young age. One of the most valuable lessons I learned from my grandmother was that our beliefs can heal us or harm us.

One thing I found out over the years is that while some home remedies have an almost instant effect on the body, some only work because people believe in them. I've seen that many times, it is the belief you have in these remedies that causes them to have an effect on the body. Most diseases stem from the mind. When unease in the body causes worry and fear in the individual, this state of mind can cause further harm to the body. For instance, there was once a man who suffered a terrible headache. To cure him, a certain woman gave him a bottle of spinach juice. She told him that the potion was a strong painkiller. Because of the woman's reputation as a known healer, the man drank the potion and immediately the pain went away. It was clear that it wasn't the spinach juice that healed the man but the man's faith in the spinach juice.

Personally, I can testify to the power of belief in my life. I have never believed in medication or drugs and each time I fall sick, I always believe that the body has the power to heal itself if nourished properly, so I take more vegetable and fruits to get better. The vegetables and fruits I take at that time are definitely not the reason I recovered, but it was my faith and belief in them that made me well.

Another event happened with a friend of mine. My friend had issues with premature ejaculation (PE). He is a person who is very health conscious and tries his best to maintain a healthy lifestyle. So, naturally speaking, he had no reasons for developing PE. He came to me for help., After speaking with him, I found out that his problems were likely to have been caused by anxiety and his mental state. I made a little concoction of honey and cinnamon for him. Although this concoction had nothing to do with premature ejaculation, I gave it to him claiming that it was a strong potion for PE. My friend believed me and took the portion. After two days he came to me saying that the potion worked wonders for him and he wished to buy more of it. At this point, I felt I had done my friend wrong, so I confessed to him that what I had given him had nothing to do with PE, and that his problems stem from his mind. I told him that he should try as much as possible not to be anxious and to go slowly during intercourse.

I have seen this type of belief work in different countries. For example, in Mexico there is a widely accepted belief that to cure a snake bite, a person should apply guaco leaves or apply tobacco on the bite . It is also said that the individual should bite a snake or smear snake bile on the bite. We all know that these remedies have no direct effect on a snake bite. But we see that they have the power to make the individuals less afraid. How it works for them is totally beyond me.

Most people are in bondage today because of their beliefs. I once heard about a particular woman who believed strongly that she was being bewitched. She sought the help of various traditional medicine men. She imagined she would be attacked with a disease by a witch, so she started to take different kinds of 'spiritual potions' to keep her protected. In a short while, she developed a big tumour on her genitals and died.

My grandmother taught me that if a person believes that he or she is being bewitched, then he or she is a victim of fear and might very well become ill one day.

The Witch has no power to harm you. All she has is her ability to make you believe that she can.

One particular day, my mom gave me a book to read. She had said it was given to her by her father, my grandfather. That book changed my life. The book was titled The Game of Life and How to Play It by Florence Scovel Shinn. If you can lay your hands on a copy, I'd suggest you buy it. I have followed the principles in that book over the years, and my life is better because of the spiritual lessons I learnt from it. This book taught me that whatever a man believes and imagines, sooner or later, will materialize in his affairs. I have always wanted to write a book that would be sold world-wide and if you are reading this book today, that imagination became a reality. So, I'm saying that a person who has trained his imagination to visualize only good things will bring into his life love, friendship, his highest ideas and everything good. In saying this, I don't mean that you will experience only good deeds and events. No, you will certainly experience the bad and heart wrecking ones, but know that those bad ones hold in them greater seeds of greatness only if we can turn our eyes away from what seem to appear wrong with the physical eyes and focus on what blessings and breakthroughs the events hold. An example of this is a time when I was sacked from my job without notice. At that moment, I chose not to focus on the bad situation but to look for the seed of greatness hidden in that event. That was the defining moment of my life. I decided to give my dreams my best shot and the idea of writing this book came. If I hadn't lost my job, you wouldn't be reading this book today, and I would never have become an author.

The book states that the mind is divided into three compartments: the subconscious, conscious and superconscious. The subconscious has no direction, and no power of deduction and whatever a man imagines clearly and holds for long in his conscious mind will be impressed into the subconscious mind which in turn will manifest in his reality. The conscious mind is the carnal mind otherwise known as the human mind. It sees our day to day life and reality, poverty, disease, suffering, and limitations and impresses these into the subconscious mind. The superconscious mind is the mind of God in all of us and within it is the realm of perfect ideas. In it lies the divine pattern or divine design for every man. Every man born on earth has a divine design, which simply refers to what he is put on earth to do. There is a position you are to fill in which no one else can and a task you should do which no one else can do. Most of us wander aimlessly through life in search of security in life while not living at all. The superconscious mind holds man's true destiny and sometimes, it flashes across the conscious mind as an unattainable goal. Therefore, it is man's duty to discover what assignment he or she is put on earth to fulfill. If this assignment is not done, man's purpose wouldn't be fulfilled on earth. Striving for material things and being covetous, can only bring us more pain and failure.

Although this book isn't meant to teach you about the spiritual laws, I feel obliged to show you how your thoughts can cause diseases in your body. Resentment, criticism, and guilt are negative thought patterns, and when held for long in the subconscious mind, they can cause diseases your body. Louis Hay in her book, You Can Heal Yourself, writes that criticism as a permanent habit can often lead to arthritis in the body. Guilt always looks for punishment, and punishment creates pain. Fear and the tension it produces can create things like baldness, ulcers, and even sore feet. Most diseases stem from a state of unforgiveness and just by forgiving and releasing resentment we can dissolve something as strong as cancer. It is very imperative for our own healing that we release the things holding us back and forgive ourselves and everyone else. To forgive and let go isn't hard. The most important thing is that we are willing to, this alone activates the healing process. To win in life, set your mind free of hate, resentment and only occupy your mind with positive thoughts. Believe in yourself, discover your life's purpose, give it your best shot and never give up. Most importantly read books, because that's the only way you will get to increase in knowledge. I love you, and I wish you well as you discover your own divine design and live a fulfilled life.

CHAPTER I

50 Marvellous Miracles of Baking Soda

Before I discovered the miracles of baking soda, a colleague at the office suffered from terrible body odour. For some reason the conventional deodorant wasn't working for him and nobody wanted to sit close to him, because once he started to sweat the air around him became contaminated. Nobody wanted to work with him on any projects., so he was at risk of losing his job. One morning, he started walking towards me. I immediately started walking in the other direction and he shouted out, "Please Marvin, I'd love to speak to you" I was tempted to pinch my nose as I walked towards him, but that would have been disrespectful. Then he said, "I visited your blog today and I see you have remedies for everything. Please can you help me?" I felt a deep compassion for this man and I made it my goal to help him solve his problem. When I got home, I went through my grandmother's journal, searching for body odour remedies. And that's when I discovered the wonders of baking soda.

Baking soda helps to absorb moisture from the skin while keeping it dry. Applying it under the arm kills bacteria and neutralizes the body to prevent excess sweating and odour. The following day I gave him this remedy and I noticed the instant look of joy and relief on his face. The following week he came back to me looking so confident, greeting everybody on his way, and speaking out loud. He told me he could never thank me enough and that he had ditched his toothpaste and house cleansers and replaced them with baking soda. I burst out laughing and gave him a hug (because he smelt good)! Baking soda is used for many other things aside from getting rid of body odour. That's what this whole book is all about. Baking soda, also known as sodium bicarbonate, helps regulate pH and keeps every substance it comes in contact with neither too acid nor too alkaline. When it comes in contact with either an acidic or alkaline substance it neutralizes its pH. So without further ado, I will now give you the fifty marvellous miracles of baking soda.

Fights Acne and Pimples:

Baking soda plays a huge role in fighting acne due to its antiseptic and anti-inflammatory properties. Baking soda is amphoteric, which gives it the ability to act as a base or acid. This characteristic helps it correct the pH imbalance of the skin that contributes to acne formation. To use baking soda as an acne remedy please follow the simple steps outlined below. to create a baking soda face mas

Directions:
- *Step 1*: First, wash your face with warm water and clean it thoroughly.
- *Step 2:* Take 6 teaspoons of sodium bicarbonate and pour it inside a container of your choice.
- *Step 3:* Add a reasonable amount of water into the container.
- *Step 4:* Use a teaspoon to stir the mixture until it's a creamy consistency.
- *Step 5:* Once smooth, apply the paste to your pimples.
- *Step 6:* Leave it on your face for about 15 minutes until the paste dries and then rinse.
- *Step 7:* Pat dry and gently clean your face with a soft hand towel.
- *Step 8:* Apply moisturizer. I prefer to use coconut oil.
- *Step 9:* Do this facial mask at least twice a week until the pimples disappear.

Teeth Whitener:

Forget the store bought teeth whiteners and the tooth paste. Nothing does the job like baking soda. I've tried it myself. Baking soda works as a mild abrasive to help remove yellow stains from the teeth, and it neutralizes the acid produced by the bacteria.

Directions:
- *Step 1:* I simply replaced my toothpaste for baking soda. Alternatively, here is a simple recipe for teeth whitener:
- *Step2:* Prepare a mixture of 4 table spoons of turmeric root powder, 2 teaspoons of baking soda, and 3 tablespoons of extra-virgin oil. Use a small amount of this mixture to brush your teeth daily. Note: Avoid excess use of baking soda as it can strip your teeth of its natural, protective enamel.

Treats Sunburn:

I've also tried this myself and I noticed it has this ability to reduce the itching and burning sensation associated with sunburn. Its mild antiseptic and drying properties help dry out sunburn blisters quickly.

Directions:
- *Step 1:* Mix 1 to 2 tablespoons of baking soda in cold water.
- *Step2:* Using a clean towel collect a reasonable amount of the mixture and gradually apply it as a cool compress on the affected area for about 7 minutes. Repeat this process two or three times a day until you feel relief.

And here's a second option: Add ½ cup of baking soda to your bathtub filled with water, stir well, and immerse yourself into the water for 10 to 15 minutes. After pat dry and then allow your body to air dry. Try this once daily for a few weeks.

Improves Skin Complexion:

Don't waste your money on store-bought creams that hardly fulfil any of the promises on their labels. Instead, choose baking soda, which is an inexpensive solution for a brighter skin tone. Baking soda is also a good exfoliating agent, which helps remove dead skin cells and balances the pH level

Directions:
- *Step 1:* Make a paste of baking soda by mixing it with water.
- *Step 2:* Apply the paste on your face and allow it to sit for at least 2 minutes.
- *Step 3:* Gently massage it while it is on your face.
- *Step 4:* When you are done, wash off with lukewarm and pat dry.

I recommend you follow this remedy at least once or twice weekly. Always remember to moisturize your skin with coconut oil after using baking soda. Apply the paste onto your face and leave for about 5 minutes. Rinse with cold water. Repeat this process two to three times a week.

Ulcer Pain:

In the past I felt down with an ulcer and I kept taking over the counter medications but the pain was severe, so a friend suggested I try baking soda. As a lover of natural remedies I didn't doubt it. I gave it a try and was surprised at how remarkably effective it was. Baking soda neutralizes stomach acid. Take 1-2 teaspoons in a glass of water and drink.

Treats Body Odour:

Baking soda works pretty well in this department if you recall the incident with my work colleague. It has a way of absorbing moisture and sweat from the skin and due to its antibacterial property it helps kill odour causing bacteria. It also lowers the pH level of the sweat glands to counteract the acids in sweat.

Directions:
- *Step 1:* Make a mixture of ½ teaspoon of baking soda, 1 tablespoon of water, and a few drops of any essential oil of your choice.
- *Step 2:* Use your fingers to take a little and gradually rub it underarm or on areas where you sweat excessively.
- Another alternative is to mix 1 tablespoon of baking soda and freshly squeezed lemon juice into a bowl and apply this under your arms. Allow it to sit for 10 minutes before you wash it off.

Removes Dandruff:

I got this tip from my mum who's a big fan of baking soda. In fact, she's so obsessed with it that she doesn't allow us (her children) to go anywhere near hers. She mostly uses it to rid her hair of dandruff. This option is also ideal for those who have an oily scalp, and suffer from the oily dandruff.

Directions:
Brace up, as I'm about to give you mum's secret recipe (please don't let her know I did)!
- *Step 1*: Mix 2 teaspoons of bicarbonate with a little water to make a paste.
- *Step 2:* Dampen your hair and rub the paste on the scalp.
- *Step 3:* Massage onto your hair thoroughly, especially on those areas which have more flaking.
- *Step 4:* After the massage, leave the mixture on your hair for about 15 minutes, then wash it off with warm water. I recommend you use this at least three times a week.
- Another great alternative is to mix lemon juice with 1 teaspoon of baking soda and apply the mixture to your scalp. Allow it to sit for 2 to 3 minutes then rinse off with warm water. Do this at least once a week, and I bet you will see remarkable results.

Treats Stained or Yellow Nails:

Do you want to whiten you nails? If so, you just bought the right book! Baking soda's bleaching and exfoliating properties helps do the job just fine.

Directions:
- **Step 1:** Mix ½ cup of water, 1 teaspoon of 3 % hydrogen peroxide, and 1 tablespoon of baking soda in a small bowl.
- **Step 2:** Stir the mixture thoroughly until the baking soda dissolves.
- **Step 3:** Then gently dip your nails into the mixture leaving them there for about 5 minutes.
- Alternatively, make a paste of baking soda and hydrogen peroxide, and use a cotton swab to apply it on your nails. Wait for about 5 minutes before rinsing your nails. You can do this once every month.

Constipation:

I know how it feels, going for days without pooping. On one occasion, I experienced severe constipation. My poops were so hard that I had to use my fingers to pull them out my anus. After I experienced minor bleeding in my anus. Later, I stumbled on an article on the web about how baking soda can help to relieve constipation. I tried it out and it worked. Baking soda is a bicarbonate and when it enters your body, it forces air to escape, which relieves some of the pain and discomfort caused by the build-up. It also acts as a mild laxative, which helps loosen bulky stools to make the passage less painful. Due to its alkaline property it helps neutralize acid and helps stored waste pass through the intestine easily.

Directions:
- **Step 1:** Add 1 teaspoon of baking soda to a glass and pour ¼ cups of warm water into it.
- **Step 2:** Stir the mixture until the baking soda is totally dissolved.
- **Step 3:** Early in the morning upon waking up drink the mixture on an empty stomach to help break down food and help it pass more easily through the colon. Make sure to consume plenty of water while on this remedy.
- Alternatively, mix 1 teaspoon of baking soda with 2 tablespoons of apple cider vinegar. Take this mixture once to twice daily depending on the severity of your symptom.

Yeast Infection:

Yeast infection is a terrible condition that affects the vagina and causes severe irritation, discharge, and intense itchiness of the vagina and vulva. No girl wants to live with this. and no guy want to be with a girl with such a condition. I've seen many girls go through this infection with no clue about how to remedy it. Some fall prey to the expensive store-bought pills. Yeast infection is usually caused by a bacteria called candida albicans. It usually exists in small quantity but an overgrowth of it may lead to an out-break of yeast infection. So how does baking soda come to the rescue? The anti-fungal property of baking soda helps to fight fungus and it can help suck the enzymes and water content from the fungus, leaving the microorganism dehydrated.

Directions:
- **Step 1:** Mix 1 tablespoon of baking soda and a pinch of sea salt into a glass of clean lukewarm water.
- **Step 2:** Then, wash the affected areas with this mixture. Repeat this process once to twice daily.
- Alternatively, mix ½ tablespoon of baking soda with 2 tablespoons of aloe vera gel. Apply this on the affected areas and leave it overnight.

Upset Stomach:

Long before I discovered the miracles of baking soda, I always grabbed the next bottle of antacids each time I experienced a queasy stomach. Thank heavens I discovered the secrets of home remedies. Baking soda is a natural antacid, which helps to neutralize the acids in your digestive tract. It also helps to break down food while making digestion easier.

Directions:
- **Step 1:** This is a simple Do It Yourself remedy I use to cure stomach upset.
- **Step 2:** Start by adding 1 teaspoon of baking soda to half a glass of water, then mix thoroughly to dissolve the solution.
- **Step 3:** Take one teaspoon every four hours. Note that this is only recommended for adults not children.
- **Step 4:** Also make sure you don't take it in large amount as it may cause high blood pressure.
- Another great alternative I recommend you try is adding 1 teaspoon of baking soda to 1 cup of warm water, then squeeze in a few drops of lemon juice. Mix thoroughly and drink. This should give you a quick relief within 10 to 15 minutes.

Diaper Rash:

I love home remedies because apart from anything else they help save money. This is good news for mothers. Instead of wasting money on expensive products, settle for a natural alternative, which is baking soda. It helps neutralize acids, balances the body's pH, and discourages the growth of yeast, bacteria, and infections.

Directions:
- *Step 1:* Simply bathe your baby's bottom in a mixture of warm water and baking soda.
- *Step 2:* You can also mix 2 – 3 tablespoons of baking soda into 3-4 cups warm water.
- *Step 3:* Then soak a clean white towel into the mixture. Use the towel to wash your baby's skin then pat dry. This should do the trick.

Insect Bites and Poison Ivy:

I can't recall how many times I've use this remedy, but it's my go-to remedy for every insect bite. Baking soda helps to relieve skin irritation and itching by neutralizing toxins and irritants in the skin surface.

Directions:
- *Step 1:* Make a paste of baking soda and water and apply to the insect bite to help relieve the itching and discomfort.
- *Step 2:* Another alternative is to rub the dry powder onto your skin. This remedy also applies to itchy rashes and poison ivy.

Heartburn, Indigestion, and Ulcer Pain:

I'm 101 per cent sure of this remedy. I've used it personally and I've also recommended it to several friends. Each of them came back with great testimonies. Baking soda neutralizes stomach acid, which helps to relieve heartburn, indigestion, and ulcer pain.

Directions:
- *Step 1:* Dissolve ½ teaspoon of baking soda in half aa glass of water and take it. (Do not take more than seven ½ teaspoons in 24 hours, or 3 ½ teaspoons if you're over 60).
- Please note that baking soda should not be taken in excess, as excessive intake can cause serious electrolyte and acid/base imbalances.

Foot Soak and Exfoliator

No one likes dry/cracked feet. This can cause severe pain and irritation whenever your feet touches the ground. It can be caused by factors such as excessively hot showers or baths, medical conditions such as diabetes or thyroid disease, low humidity levels in home, soaps that are non-moisturizing, and ageing.

Directions:
- *Step 1:* Simply add 3 tablespoons to a tub of warm water to make an invigorating foot soak.
- Alternatively, make a paste of baking soda and scrub your feet with it.

Relaxing Soak:

Looking for the best homemade relaxing soak? Venture no further! Baking soda and apple cider vinegar makes an amazing spa-like bath for soaking away aches and pains and detoxing. It doesn't stop there either! It also cleans the bath.

Enhanced Sports Performance:

You will be amazed with this. That simple white powder in your kitchen is the performance secret of most athletes. Popularly known as soda-doping amongst professional sportsmen, it has a significant effect on their endurance and speed. A study conducted at the Loughborough University found that out of nine swimmers who took baking soda before an event, eight reduced their times. How does this work? Sodium bicarbonate is alkaline in nature, which seems to increase the pH level of the blood, thereby offsetting the acidity produced in the muscles during intense, anaerobic exercise that produces lactic acid most quickly, such as fast running or swimming.

Splinter Remover:

To remove a splinter make a baking soda paste by combining baking soda and water. Apply the mixture on to the splinter then cover it up with a bandage. Leave overnight. The paste will make the splinter adhere to the bandage so it can easily come off.

Hand Cleanser:

Baking soda makes the perfect hand cleanser. For what it's worth, it's the only hand cleanser I use in my home.

Directions:
- *Step 1:* Simply mix three parts baking soda with one part water to make a natural hand cleanser that's very effective in scrubbing away dirt. It also neutralizes odour.

Remove Blackheads:

Most beauty remedies call for baking soda, so it shouldn't be much of a surprise to discover that baking soda is effective in removing blackheads. It exfoliates your skin, leaving it soft and supple while unclogging pores containing dead skin. Baking soda also neutralizes your skin pH level while making sure it produces less oil.

Directions:
- *Ss*Wash your face thoroughly with warm water to help open up the skin pores.
- *Step 2:* Then apply a paste of baking soda and water on the affected areas. Leave it for about 5 minutes, then massage your face in a circular motion to help loosen the dead skin cells, blackheads, dirt and other impurities.
- *Step 3:* Rinse with warm water.
- Alternatively, prepare a mixture of 3 tablespoons of baking soda with 3 table spoons of apple cider vinegar. While mixing, gently pour in the vinegar into the baking soda to keep the mixture from bubbling over. Then apply mixture to affected areas and leave for about 20 minutes until it is totally dry. Then rinse thoroughly with warm water.

Sweeten Your Tomatoes:

Do you know you can sweeten your tomatoes by simply sprinkling baking soda on the soil around your tomato plants? Baking soda absorbs into the soil and lowers its acidity levels giving you sweet tasting tomatoes. Don't take my word for it. Try it yourself.

Canker Sore:

Baking soda works fine with canker sores. I've tried it several times and can testify to that. It helps neutralize the acidity in your mouth while soothing the pain associated with canker sores. Baking soda anti-septic and antibacterial property helps kill bacteria and germs associated with canker sores while lessening the ability of bacteria to get into the salivary glands. Baking soda also has anti-inflammatory properties that help reduce swelling and inflammation of the mouth sores.

Directions:
- *Step 1:* Take a small amount of baking soda with your fingers and apply it directly on the canker sore.
- *Step 2:* Leave it to sit for an hour, as this helps to neutralize and ease the pain caused by canker sore.
- *Step 3:* Finally, swish your mouth thoroughly with warm water and spit out. Repeat this twice daily, and your canker sore will gradually vanish.
- Alternatively, you can use hydrogen peroxide and baking soda. Hydrogen peroxide has anti-bacterial and antiseptic properties that help kill bacteria and reduce the inflammation. Combined with baking soda it gives a rapid result. Make a solution of hydrogen peroxide and baking soda, swish your mouth thoroughly with the solution at least four to five times a day. Repeat this until the canker sore has totally gone.

Great Scrub:

Looking for the best bath and kitchen scrub? Try baking soda, as it's highly effective in that department. To create a handy scrub simply pour baking soda in a glass grated cheese container with a stainless top that has holes in it. Use it to sprinkle the baking soda on the surface and scrub.

Pamper Your Feet:

Give your feet a treat by soaking them in a baking soda solution to soothe and soften. To do this, mix 4 tablespoons of baking soda in a small tub of warm water and soak your feet in it.

Freshen Sponges:

To get rid of that smell in your sponge, mix 4 tablespoons of baking soda in 1 quart of warm water. Then soak the sponge into the solution to get rid of the smell.

Deodorize Garbage Disposals:

I usually get irritating odour from down sink drainage. I stopped this by pouring baking soda solution down skin drainage. The odour stopped immediately.

Get rid of Toilet Odour:

I love this particular one, as it's very effective. I do it almost all the time. My toilet comes out sparkling and odourless. Simply sprinkle baking soda inside your toilet and leave it for an hour before scrubbing.

Carpet Deodorizer:

Although this process can be a little bit tedious, it works. Sprinkle baking soda on your carpet and let it sit overnight. In the morning sweep them off and perhaps also use a vacuum.

Dry Shampoo:

Are you still spending a fortune on dry shampoo? You will be pleased to know that baking soda does the job. Sprinkle a little baking soda at the root of your hair, especially in the areas that tend to get oily, then use your fingers to distribute it. Let it sit for about 10 minutes so it can absorb the oil. Then comb the excess shampoo out of your hair. Turn your hair upside down and brush out the powder. I suggest you use a hair dryer to help you with this.

Volumizing Shampoo:

You can add volume to your hair by mixing a quarter size of baking soda to your daily dollop of shampoo. This helps to remove impurities, leaving your hair lighter and with a full on volume.

Cleaning Agent:

When a hairbrush is used over a long period of time it gets dirty and oily. You can keep it neat and dirt free by placing it in a bowl of warm water mixed with 3 tablespoons of baking soda.

Facial Scrub:

This is my mum's favourite scrub recipe. She adds a tablespoon of baking soda to her facial cleanser to form a paste. She then massages it onto her face in a circular motion. Doing this leaves her skin feeing soft.

Nail Cleaner:

To get rid of the yellowish stain on your nails due to some excessive applications of nail polish, mix baking soda and hydrogen peroxide and scrub it on your nails.

Smelly Shoes:

Do you have smelly shoes? Then just sprinkle baking soda in your shoes for a natural deodorizer.

Remove Chlorine from Hair:

If you love swimming as much as I do, chances aree you might have some chlorine build up in your hair. To get rid of this, mix baking soda with dish soap and apply onto your hair. Leave it to sit for 10 minutes and wash off with warm water. Then condition your hair.

Pedicure:

Give yourself a spa pedicure at home. Mix 2 to 3 tablespoons of baking soda with water for a soothing foot soak. Add your favourite essential oil (such as lavender oil) and soak for 20 minutes. Then scrub your feet with a paste of baking soda and water to help exfoliate rough spots.

Modelling Clay:

You can easily turn baking soda into modelling clay by combining it with one and 1/4 cups of water and one cup of cornstarch.

Natural Oven Cleaning:

Still looking for the most effective oven cleaner? Try baking soda. Simply sprinkle baking soda on the bottom of the oven, spray or sprinkle with water until it forms a paste, and leave for several hours. Stuck on grease and burnt on food wipes right off.

Soften Fabric:

Baking soda can also be used as a fabric softener in your laundry, or to get your clothes whiter and brighter. I do this frequently for my white t-shirts. Sart by adding one cup to your laundry load.

Silver Polish:

I got this tip from the Dr. Mercola website and I think it's worth trying. To polish silver without using toxic silver polish, fill your kitchen sink with hot water, add a sheet of aluminum foil, and baking soda, and let the silver pieces soak until they're clean. It is an easy and fun way to clean silver.

Clean Kitchen Utensils:

To clean out your pots and pans from debris of baked food, soak them in hot water and baking soda. Leave it for about 15 minutes, and the stain will come off easily.

Air freshener:

I still have two bottles remaining from the one I did last week (As at the time this book was written) Most air fresheners in the market are full of toxic chemicals that shouldn't pass through the nostrils. I discovered a simple DIY air freshener that calls for baking soda.

Neutralize Gassy Beans:

The only reason I disliked eating beans was the constant gassing. It can cause huge embarrassment when the gas is smelly. But when I discovered that baking soda can help with this, I rekindled my love for beans. To do this sprinkle a teaspoon of baking soda in water when you soak your beans to prevent gassy issues and improve digestion.

Produce Wash:

I'm a huge juicing enthusiast. Sometimes it's hard to get organic produce, but when you settle for non-organic once, you have to make sure it's properly washed. A mixture of baking soda and water does the job perfectly for me.

Keep Ants Out:

To keep ants out, mix equal parts of baking soda and salt together. Sprinkle the mixture wherever you see the ants, and they will do a "U turn."

Erase Crayon, Pencil, Ink, and Furniture Scuffs from Painted Surfaces:

Sprinkle baking soda onto a slightly wet towel and rub lightly, then wipe off with a clean, dry cloth.

Deodorize Garbage Cans:

To do this, sprinkle some baking soda on the bottom of your trash cans to help keep bad smells away.

Boiling Chicken:

When boiling a chicken, add a teaspoon of baking soda to the water. The feathers will come off easier, and the flesh will be clean and white.

Keep Flowers Fresher Longer:

Baking soda is also used in keeping flowers fresh. Simply add 1 tablespoon to the water in the flower vase.

CHAPTER 2

Amazing Benefits of Enemas

Have you ever thought about cleansing your colon? I guess not, but it might interest you to know that the average person walks around daily with 3 to 7 pounds of fecal materials in their large intestine. That's kind of gross, but it's a fact.

Most of the time, due to our uber-unhealthy lifestyle, our bowel becomes sluggish or constipated and this leads to fecal matters being deposited along the walls of the colon, which can lead to inflammation. Over time the matter begins to decay and releases harmful toxins into the organs, which have dire effects on the absorption of nutrients and may lead to other illnesses. It's true that many chronic health conditions can be treated with enemas. With all the hype about enemas, you might be wondering what the heck an enema is. In simple terms an enema happens when you inject enough filtered water into your colon to stimulate peristalsis throughout your entire colon.

This singular action helps to clean the entire large intestine. Once you have enough water in your colon, visit the toilet and force out the resulting waste. There are various kinds of enema but a coffee enema is the most popular.

Coffee Enema The coffee enema is prepared by brewing organic caffeinated beans and letting the brew cool to body temperature, then delivering it via an enema bag. It contains choleretics, a substance that increases the flow of toxins-rich bile to the gallbladder. A coffee enema is the best ways to help speed up our body's healing process by causing the liver to deposit its toxic waste within seconds into the intestines to be removed from the body via the poop or faeces. This process is so important because dead tumours collect in the liver and have the potential to kill the patient if the liver can't get rid of them fast enough. The coffee enema was extensively used in the 1940's by Dr. Max Gerson in the treatment plan of his cancer patients.

The Amazing Health Benefits of Coffee Enemas:

- The coffee enema enhances digestion by increasing bile flow and removes toxins in the large intestine. Most people have viscous unhealthy bile due to a long history of unhealthy lifestyles, and toxins in their environments. Coffee enemas are the best way to have a thin and healthy free-flowing bile. Coffee enemas help the liver release bile. When the flow of bile is enhanced, the liver can remove toxins and poisons more effectively.

- Coffee also acts as an astringent in the large intestine, helping to clean the colon walls. The use of a coffee enema helps rid the body of toxins. Over time the process helps to create a healthier environment in the colon and enhances bowel function in the body.

- Coffee enemas are particularly helpful for slow oxidizers. Their liver activity is more sluggish and digestion is usually impaired. Fast oxidizers may have more difficulty retaining the enema. It also increases the body's ability to produce glutathione, the major liver antioxidant, which helps bind with toxins and usher them out of the body during an enema session.

- Coffee enemas can heal chronic health conditions, along with following a raw food plan.

- Coffee enemas Increase energy levels while improving mental clarity and mood.

- Coffee enhances the elimination of toxins through the liver. Indeed, endoscopic studies confirm they increase bile output, and less toxins stuck in the body allows for a healthier colon which can maintain healthy gut bacteria.

Procedures:

The first thing you need to do is purchase an enema kit. This kit can be purchased on Amazon. There are two options to choose from; either a traveller's kit or a bucket type kit.

- Purchase your premium ground coffee beans and store them in the refrigerator.
- Pour 2 tablespoons of organic coffee in the saucepan and add 3 cups of distilled water.
- Boil the mixture and let it simmer for at least 15 minutes.
- Remove from heat and cool.
- Strain the mixture with a mesh strainer or nut milk bag into a clean glass pouring jar.
- Visit the toilet and set up a space comfortable for you to lie on.
- Next set up your enema kit. It should come with a tube and nozzle attached to the bucket or bag (make sure it's at least 1 meter above the ground).
- Take a closer look at the enema bag/bucket, and make sure the clamp that allows you control the flow of coffee is set to off before pouring the coffee into the bag.
- After pouring the coffee into the bag, hold the tube and nozzle over your shower plug and turn it on.
- Get rid of the air by allowing the coffee to run through the tube, then stop the flow afterwards.
- Lubricate the nozzle with olive oil for ease of insertion.
- Lie down on your right side with your knees drawn up.
- Insert the nozzle into the rectum about 1 inch deep.
- Turn on the flow of coffee slowly and gently squeeze the bag until it is empty.
- Lie on your back with your feet resting on a wall above head level.
- If you hear some squirting noises in the stomach, that's a good sign that the bile is being stimulated for release.

- Retain the enema for 12 to 15 minutes. A strong urge may arise to go to the toilet. Try to hold on for as long as you can until the sensation eases.
- Head to the toilet and let it go. Don't forget to keep your enema clean before packing it away.

It's recommended that patients with chronic diseases should take enemas six times daily and those on detox programs or cleansing should limit it to once daily until the end of their program. During a healing reaction, two enemas daily should be taken. For those who are very ill, several a day may be best for at least several months. The best time to take the enema is after a normal bowel movement. Coffee enemas should not be taken in the evening because it might interfere with sleep.

Epsom Salt Enema:

Epsom salt can be found in most pharmacies and is used to increase the amount of water absorbed by the intestine, producing a laxative effect, which results in thorough cleansing of the intestinal tract. This makes it highly effective in colon cleansing. They are commonly used to relieve pain caused by arthritis, but can be taken internally as an enema for constipation relief. An Epsom salt enema is a faster way to get results than when taken orally.

Epsom Salt Enema Recipe:
- 4 tbsp. Epsom salts
- 2 qts. warm water
- Enema bag with tube
- IV stand
- Lubricant

Procedure:

- Mix 2 tablespoons of Epson salt with 2 quarts of warm water.
- Stir the mixture thoroughly until the salt is completely dissolved.
- Fill the Epsom salt into the enema bag and hang over the IV stand.
- Place your knees and hands on the ground, lowering your chest to the floor.
- Keep your anus as high as possible.
- Insert the lubricated enema tub into your anus.
- Allow the enema solution to enter your colon slowly.
- Leave until the bag is empty.
- Use one hand to massage your abdomen in a clockwise direction to evenly distribute the solution throughout the colon.
- Retain the same position and hold the enema in the colon for about 3 to 5 minutes for a proper cleanse.
- Move to the toilet and release the enema. Cautions and Considerations:
- If you have stomach pain, nausea, or vomiting, please do not administer the Epsom enema.

Excessive or improper use of Epsom salts can result in hypomagnesaemia, so keep the dosage to 300-400 milligrams daily.

Lemon Juice Enema

A Lemon Juice Enema helps rid the colon of excess faeces and balances the pH level in the colon. This enema can also help relieve chronic constipation and pain associated with colitis. It generally produces mild irritation to the intestinal lining. A lemon juice enema will help balance the pH factor in your colon.

Enema Recipe:
- 1/3 cup real-lemon (unsweetened lemon juice) per quart
- 2 quarts of warm filtered water
- Enema bag with tube
- IV stand
- Lubricant

Procedure:

- Mix the 1/3 cup of lemon juice to 2qts of warm filtered water.
- Add the solution to the enema bag. Hang the enema bag about 18inch to 3ft above your rectum using the IV stand.
- Use the ramp clamp to get a good flow for the enema solution.
- Place your knees and hands on the ground, lowering your chest to the floor.
- Keep your anus as high as possible.
- Insert the lubricated enema tub into your anus.
- Allow the enema solution to enter your colon slowly.
- Leave till the bag is empty.
- You can refill the bag if needed and if you experience cramping because the solution is cool, stop the flow for a few seconds until the cramps subside.
- Then restart the enema.
- Massaging the abdomen in a counter-clockwise direction during the injection will distribute the solution throughout the colon.
- Retain the solution for several minutes a this will allow the enema to do its job. If you have a problem retaining the enema for a longer period, I suggest you fold a washcloth and press it tightly against your anus, or use a retention plug. Then you can move to the toilet and release the enema.

Salt Water Enema

The salt water enema is the most common enema you can use. It helps reduce the absorption of water into the bloodstream. This process prevents filling your kidney and bladder with water. Salt reduces the amount of water absorbed into the bloodstream, so you will also experience less need for urination while holding this enema, and it makes for effective softening old fecal impaction.

Enema Recipe:
- 2 tsp pure sea salt
- 2 litres of water Procedure
- Enema bag with tube
- IV stand
- Lubricant

Procedure:

- Add the mixture to an enema bag.
- Hang the enema bag about 18 in. to 3 ft. above your rectum using the IV Stand for enemas.
- If you need good flow control for the enema solution use a ramp clamp.
- Place your knees and hands on the ground, lowering your chest to the floor.
- Keep your anus as high as possible. Insert the lubricated enema tub into your anus.
- Allow the enema solution to enter your colon slowly.
- Leave until the bag is empty.
- You can refill the bag if needed.
- If you experience some cramping because the solution is cool, stop the flow for a few seconds until the cramps subside. Then restart the enema.
- Retain the solution for several minutes as, this will allow the enema to do its job. Then you can move to the toilet and release the enema.

Acidophilus Enema

This type of enema is mostly recommended for those suffering from irritable bowel syndrome, constipation, inflammatory bowel disease, haemorrhoids or colon cancer. It is well known for its ability to replenish beneficial bacteria when administered directly into the colon.

Enema Recipe:
- 4 tablespoons live culture yogurt or
- 4 - 5 capsules dry acidophilus or
- 1 tsp. powdered acidophilus
- 2 quarts warm filtered water (mix well)
- Enema bag with tube
- IV stand
- Lubricant

Procedure:

- Start by adding acidophilus, mixed with warm water into an enema bag.
- Hang the enema bag about 18 in. to 3 ft. above your rectum using the IV Stand for Enemas. For a better flow control, use the ramp clamp.
- Place your knees and hands on the ground, lowering your chest to the floor.
- Keep your anus as high as possible.
- Insert the lubricated enema tub tip into your anus (using a good lubricant will help prevent injury to delicate anal tissues.)
- Allow the enema solution to enter your colon slowly. Leave until the bag is empty.
- Feel free to refill the bag if you wish, until it becomes very uncomfortable to take any more solution.
- I advise you massage your abdomen in a counter-clockwise direction during injection, as this helps the solution reach higher into the colon.
- When you notice you are no longer capable of taking any more fluid, remove the nozzle. If you have trouble retaining the solution, you can use a washcloth and press it tightly against the anus.
- You can now move to the toilet and release the enema. While releasing the enema, massage the abdomen to help move the solution back towards the rectum and anus.

CHAPTER 3

Sure-fire Ways to Lose Weight in Ten Days

Losing weight is not as hard as people make it look. I guess most people search for quick fixes, like one of my friends, David. David is borderline line obese and he wouldn't heed any of my advice when it came to weight loss. David would rather invest in fake pills that promise weight loss than live a healthy lifestyle. However, after taking these pills for the last three years he is still gaining more weight. He is now considering liposuction.

If you aren't very active in the day and would love to lose weight, then your diet is key. Try to avoid eating junk foods. I know junk food can be tempting but discipline yourself and say no to such foods. When you take junk food into your body, you are putting more calories into your body than it needs. These foods contain large quantities of sugar, sodium, unhealthy fats, all of which promote weight gain. If you're really serious about your weight loss goals stick to food such as lean meat, fruits, vegetables, whole grains, and healthy fats. These foods are low in calories and contain nutrients that help you build lean muscle and promote healthy digestion, in turn leading to weight loss. Secondly, eat smaller meals more frequently, but make sure they are healthy meals. Portioning your meals like this helps keep your metabolism higher enabling you to burn more calories. Eating more often also ensures that your blood sugar levels stay normal and stops you from over eating. To achieve this I suggest you stick to 200 to 300 calories meals eaten two to three hours apart Remember, it's not just about eating smaller meals frequently. You also need to spread out the nutrients with each meal you eat. For instance, eating too many carbohydrates with a particular meal can lead to fat storage, while eating too much protein can lead to constipation. According to the National Strength and Conditioning Association, you should aim to eat 20 per cent to 35 per cent of your daily calories from protein; 45 per cent to 65 per cent from carbohydrates; and about 15 per cent to 25 per cent from healthy fats. Apply these ratios to each meal to ensure proper nutrient intake. Some foods that can help you lose weight are Hot Peppers, Green Tea, Whole Grains, Quinoa and Oats, Grapefruit and other Citrus Fruits, Lean Poultry and Fish, Beans and Lentils, Berries, Apples, Almonds, Almond, Milk and Almond Butter, Eggs, Greek Yogurt, Spinach, and Broccoli. Another important consideration is how much water you are drinking. Water has a huge role to play in our overall health and weight loss and its best to drink hot water than cold water because hot water stays in your stomach longer than cold water and makes you feel fuller, helping to reduce your cravings. Researchers in Germany report that water consumption increases the rate at which people burn calories. Water helps facilitate the metabolic process, which in turns help you burn calories. Try to drink about eight 8-ounce glasses of water per day to stay hydrated.

Cinnamon:

Abdominal fat is a huge problem area for many people. The good news is that the consumption of cinnamon helps burn fat, especially in that region. Cinnamon imitates the activity of insulin in the body, which helps the body regulate its blood sugar level. Maintaining blood sugar level is very important for weight loss. Cinnamon also produces heat through metabolic situations, which helps you burn fat. Please note that ground cinnamon should be taken rather than the bark oil. The bark oil may lead to ulcers, mouth sores and mouth burning when consumed.

Usage:

- Always add ground cinnamon to your beverages.
- Use cinnamon to toast your muffins by adding it on top.
- Sprinkle grounded cinnamon on your salads, dips or sauces.
- *Alternatively* add 2 teaspoons of cinnamon to boiling water, and allow it to sit for about 10 minutes. Add a tea bag to it and drain the mixture afterward. Add honey and drink. This should be taken twice daily to prevent fat storage on your waistline.

Honey and Cinnamon:

The honey and cinnamon recipe is as old as the hills when it comes to weight loss. My grandmother used to prescribe it back in the days. I wrote about it in great detail in the chapter about the uses of honey. Honey has a healthy glycerine index that doesn't get absorbed into the body all at once like sugar. Cinnamon contributes immensely to weight loss by improving the function of insulin, stabilizes high blood pressure, boosts metabolism, and detoxifies and increases the energy levels in the body.

You need:
- Honey (1 tbsp)
- Cinnamon (1 tbsp)

Directions:
- Start by adding the cinnamon to a cup of boiling water.
- Leave it for about 15 minutes and then remove from the heat.
- Let it cool for a while, and then add honey to the water.
- Drink this mixture daily.

Always remember to add honey when the mixture it cooled, because honey tends to lose an ample amount of enzymes when added to hot water.

Lemon Juice:

A glass of lemon juice contains less than 25 calories and it's a rich source of calcium, potassium, vitamin c, and peptic fibre. Warm lemon water is the perfect "good morning drink," which helps eliminate waste products from the body. Lemon rids your body of toxins and flushes out unnecessary fat. It also prevents problems of constipation and diarrhea by ensuring smooth bowel functions.

You Need:
- 1 lemon
- 1 glass of warm water

Directions:
- First thing in the morning upon waking up, squeeze lemon juice into a glass of lukewarm water and drink it on an empty stomach. •
- Do not take any solid food for the next 45 minutes.

Water Therapy:

Water therapy is one of the most convenient and best ways to lose weight. I've tried it myself and I noticed a significant amount of change on my overall wellbeing, not only concerning weight loss. But do keep in mind that this therapy is dependent on the person's actual weight. The amount of water consumed daily must be half of the person's actual weight. If you weigh 100 pounds, then you have to consume about 50 ounces of water. Upon waking up early in the morning, before brushing your teeth, drink about 400-600 millilitres of clean water and wait for an hour before eating breakfast. If you do this for about a month you will begin to see a dramatic improvement in your overall health and weight.

Honey & Ginger Remedy:

I can't overemphasize the potency of this remedy when it comes to weight loss. If you're keen to lose weight take note of this remedy. Honey produces a natural form of sugar known as fructose. Fructose serves as a fuel for the liver to produce glucose, which signals the release of fat burning hormones in your body. Ginger is a natural appetite suppressant, which helps reduce unhealthy food cravings and boosts the metabolism.

You need:
- 3 tablespoons of honey
- 2 tablespoons of ginger

Directions:
- Start by extracting your ginger juice with a juicer.
- Add 3 tablespoons into a cup and follow it up with 3 tablespoons of honey.
- Mix thoroughly and drink this concoction twice daily.

- Within a month you will start seeing changes in your body.

Lemon, Honey, Pepper Remedy:

There's a natural weight loss clinic near where I live. On one particular occasion they advertised a secret weight loss potion they sold for over $50. I was curious to see this recipe, but I couldn't justify paying that amount, so I devised a means to get it by canvassing with one of the staff members who I knew. Finally, when this recipe was in my hands, I wasn't so thrilled and thank God I didn't pay for it. But for what it's worth, the recipe is very potent and it's widely used by Indians for weight loss. Black pepper contains piperine, which prevents the formation of new fat cells in the body and reduces the fat lenses in the blood stream. Lemon, on the other hand, helps to stabilize the body's pH level. It also contains pectin fiber, which helps prevent hunger pangs. Combining these ingredients makes for a potent weight loss potion.

You need:
- A glass of lukewarm water
- 1 tablespoon of honey
- 1 tablespoon of black pepper
- 4 tablespoons of lemon juice

Directions:
Start by heating a cup of hot water. Remove from the heat and leave it to cool. Then add 1 tablespoon of honey, 1 tablespoon of black pepper and 4 tablespoons of lemon juice. Mix thoroughly Drink the mixture first thing upon waking up every morning.

Hot Pepper:

Hot pepper can help you lose an immense amount of belly fat. Pepper contains a compound known as capsaicin, which boosts your body's heat production. Researchers from the University of California in Los Angeles tested the compound capsaicin to see if it can actually burn fat by heating the body. The result showed that it caused an increase in the number of calories burnt. When these capsinoids are taken daily, it will greatly reduce abdominal fat and improve fat oxidation. Some peppers are definitely hotter than others, with Habanero pepper being at the top of the list with the highest amount of capsaicin. Cayenne pepper also has a good amount of capsaicin, which can greatly increase the fat burning process.

How to use Hot Pepper:

- Add raw, cooked, dried or powdered pepper to your soup
- Or include habanero pepper or cayenne pepper in your diet to increase the fat burning process.

Almonds:

Studies conducted by a group of researchers led by Michelle Wien, Dr. P.H., R.D show that almonds help with weight loss. Almonds can help suppress your cravings and make you feel fuller. They contain monounsaturated fat, protein, and fiber, which also contributes to minimizing hunger pangs. Almond prevents fats and calories from being absorbed by your body, and contains oleic acid, a monounsaturated fat helping to decrease the body's cholesterol levels. A particular study shows that people who ate at least an ounce of almonds daily were found to have their LDL cholesterol level dramatically decreased, which lowers the risk of incurring heart-related conditions.

How to use almonds:
- Immerse a handful of almonds in water and leave them overnight. Eat the soaked almonds very early in the morning. Repeat this daily to get rid of stomach fat.
- You can also include almonds in your breakfast, or add them to your juices or smoothies. Or simply chew a handful of almonds daily.

Apple Cider Vinegar and Water

Apple cider vinegar is a rich source of pectin, and when included in your diet it helps make you feel fuller and more satisfied. It also helps lower blood sugar and insulin levels, so it makes total sense that it might also help with weight loss. It's a known fact that acids help with the digestion of protein, which is the building blocks for the growth hormone. Likewise the hormone helps in breaking down of fat cells. So by increasing the acid in your stomach before meals you will make room for thorough digestion and increase the availability of protein for hormone synthesis. Greater protein utilization helps the formation of growth hormones, the substance that keeps the body's metabolism going while the body is at rest. This is why it's advisable to drink apple cider vinegar before each meal. On the other hand, lemon is rich in vitamin C and has been shown to greatly aid in weight loss. Lemons promote your body's production of digestive enzymes by the liver.

You need:

- 1 bottle of water
- Apple cider vinegar
- Lemon juice

Directions:

- Start by adding one tablespoon of apple cider vinegar to a cup of water, followed by one tablespoon of lemon juice.
- Drink this concoction at least once a day for best results.

Lemon Juice and Hot Water

Many people have had great results with hot lemon and water. My mum can testify to that as she lost am ample amount of weight by following this simple remedy first thing every morning for a period of one month. Hot lemon water comes with a powerful agent that improves your chances of weight loss. This recipe's potency can be attributed to vitamin C and antioxidants of lemon coupled with the digestion improving ability of hot water. This combination helps stimulate the digestive process, and drinking warm water will slightly raise your body heat, allowing for a slight increase in thermogenesis, the process your body uses to burn calories from the foods you eat. Also, lemons are diuretic, which means they help to get rid of water weight. Drinking this concoction with a meal will also stimulate the production of gastric juices to get a head start on digesting your food. On the other hand, hot water has been widely advocated as a laxative, which helps relieve constipation by helping you pass softer stools.

You need:

- One bottle of water
- Lemon juice

Directions:

Start by warming up your water and allow it to cool to a bearable temperature. Then squeeze the juice of a fresh lemon into the hot water and drink it.

Dandelion Remedy:

There are several claims that dandelion extract can be used to achieve weight loss. These claims are mainly because of its diuretic effect and getting rid of water weight. Drinking a cup of dandelion tea before meals promotes fat and cholesterol breakdown in your body while stimulating secretions. It's also important to know that dandelion extract does not increase fat metabolism or thermogenesis, and this makes its weight loss claims a little weak. Combined with some fat reducing spices, dandelion tea not only tastes good but helps reduce belly fat, which is due to water retention.

Ingredients:
- Dandelion root (roasted) 1 tbsp OR dandelion root powder (roasted) 1 tsp
- Fresh ginger (minced)
- Cardamom seeds from 1 cardamom
- Cinnamon bark, half inch piece
- Mint leaves, 4-5
- 1 cup of water

Directions:
- Put all the ingredients in a bowl of water.
- Place the bowl of water over the heat and bring it to the boil for about 10 minutes.
- Strain the tea and drink. You can add honey if you wish. You can drink two to four cups a day.

Cabbage:

There are several claims that cabbage can be used to burn fat, but are these claims really true? The truth is that cabbage will not burn fat from your body, but it is still ideal for achieving weight loss because it's low in calories. One important reason why people associate cabbage with weight loss is due to the presence of tartaric acid. Tartaric acid prevents sugar and carbohydrates from being converted into fat in the body. Personally, I hate eating cabbage raw, but I get a lot of raw cabbage in my diet through juicing. You can also add raw cabbage to your salad or smoothies.

Hot Water Remedy:

Switching from cold water to hot water can really help your weight loss goals. Hot water stays in your stomach for a bit longer than cold water and cold water is absorbed a little bit faster than hot water. When you drink a cup of hot water you will feel fuller for a bit longer than if you drink the same amount of cold water. This remedy is helpful if you are trying to avoid snacking and over eating. Personally, I've observed that drinking hot water helps me go through the day without consuming unnecessary calories. Hot water also flushes out fats from your vessels, which in turn helps you to lose weight.

Cucumber Remedy:

I added cucumber to the list because cucumber contains 90 per cent water content and 13.25 calories. Cucumber is rich in vitamin A, C, and E, which helps eliminate toxins from the body. If your goal is to lose weight I suggest you include cucumber in your diet, which helps you lower your calorie intake and shed pounds. A medium peeled cucumber has just 24 calories, while a large unpeeled cucumber has just 45 calories. Since cucumbers are this low in calories it makes perfect sense that including them in your diet is beneficial for weight loss, because they will fill you up when you are following a calorie-controlled diet.

Green Tea:

Green tea is another well-known remedy for weight loss. It contains about 25 milligrams of caffeine per 8 ounces. Caffeine found in green tea is partly responsible for its weight loss effects. It also aids in weight loss by reducing your appetite and boosting metabolism. Also, the compound epigallocatechin-3-gallate found in green tea helps prevent weight gain and obesity by limiting the absorption of fat and enhancing the body's capacity to use fat for energy that is required to carry out various functions. You can have three to four cups of green daily for weight loss. Below is a simple fat burning green tea you can try.

Ingredients:
- Green tea leaves or green tea bag
- 1 cup of hot water
- 4-5 mint/basil leaves
- 1 tablespoon of lemon juice
- 1 – 2 tablespoons of Honey

Directions:
- Start by adding green tea and mint leaves into a cup or bowl of boiling water.
- Remove from the heat and leave it to steep for about 5 – 10 minutes.
- Strain the mixture and add lemon juice plus honey.
- Drink three to four cups daily after meals.

Garlic and Lemon Remedy

You might already know that garlic is good for your cardiovascular system as it reduces both systolic and diastolic blood pressure, as well as triglycerides, apart from increasing good cholesterol. You might, however, not know that garlic has excellent anti-obesity properties too. Every minute our body cells die and our body makes new cells to replace them. Adipocytes (also called lipocytes and fat cells) are the cells in our body which primarily compose adipose tissue (body fat). In the adipose tissue there undergoes a process where pre-adipocytes are converted into full-fledged adipose tissue or fat. This process is known as adipogenesis. Studies show that garlic inhibits this process of adipogenisis or the process of making fat. In simple language, garlic stops your pre-fat cells from converting into fat cells. So, you might like to add garlic into your daily diet. However, raw garlic is more beneficial when you want to lose belly fat.

Get this:
- 3 Garlic cloves
- 1 Lemon
- 1 cup Water

Do this:
- Squeeze the lemon juice into the cup of water and add the juice of garlic clove into the lemon water.
- Drink the resulting mixture. Repeat this every morning on an empty stomach.
- You will start losing belly fat within two weeks.

Cranberry Juice:

Cranberry juice can help you burn belly fat by boosting your metabolism. Cranberries are high in organic acid, which acts as digestive enzymes. These enzymes help flush out fat deposits that get stuck in the lymphatics. Cranberry juice also helps prevent various infections of the bladder and helps to increase the overall energy levels of the body.

You need:
- Cranberry juice
- 7 ounces of water

Directions:
- Mix one ounce of pure cranberry juice with 7 ounces of water.
- Drink this mixture very early in the morning on an empty stomach.
- Alternatively, you can add lemon juice to the mixture to speed up the fat burning process.

Coconut Oil

Yes, it's true, coconut oil can really help you lose those unwanted fats, but definitely not by eating it. Rather by substituting it with other fats. Unlike most other saturated fats, coconut oil doesn't get packed away as fat. It is sent straight to the liver to be metabolized, giving you an energy boost. This energy makes exercising easier, which in turn helps you to lose weight. It also acts as an appetite suppressant. Just by taking 2 teaspoons of coconut oil, you can greatly reduce your cravings. Coconut oil is also a thermogenic, which means that it heats up the body internally and helps to burn fat. A particular study was conducted in reducing abdominal fat where a group of women were divided into two groups. One group were given 2 teaspoons of coconut oil for a period of 28 days, while the other group were given soybeans oil for the same amount of days. Both groups lost 2 pounds but the group fed with coconut oil reduced their waistline while the other group had a mild increase of belly fat.

How to use coconut oil to reduce belly fat:
- Replace other oil you use daily with coconut oil •Minimize your intake of coconut oil to 2 tablespoons a day
- Incorporate a whole food diet to your lifestyle, along with coconut oil.

Omega-3 Fatty Acids:

If you really want to burn belly fat then omega-3 / fish oil is highly recommended as it helps break down fat around the waistline. You can either take 6g of the supplement or eat salmon or mackerel twice a week. For a rapid result, I suggest you add chia seeds to the mix. These seeds are high in protein, calcium, antioxidants, and it's a good source of vitamin B.

Material Needed:
- 6g of fish oil
- Fish Directions:
- Take 6g of fish oil daily to lose belly fat
- Alternatively, eat fish such as salmon, tuna, halibut or mackerel twice weekly.

Juice Fast:

Juice fasting is another great way to lose weight. Juice fasting simply means consuming nothing but green juice for a particular amount of days. It's best to stick to vegetables if your goal is to lose weight, because fruit contains natural sugar called fructose, which can spike your sugar level. However, you can still include citrus fruits, such as lemons and apples. There are some rules you need to note before beginning a juice fast. To do a juice fast you need a juicer (a masticating juicer or twin gear juicer is preferable because those kind of juicers do well with vegetables). Juice fasts not only help you lose weight but also help in cleansing and detoxifying your body and nourishing it with the required antioxidants.

Herbal Cleanse:

This herbal treatment is very effective and I usually recommend this to my clients who are undergoing a juice fast programme. This herbal cleanse is very effective for weight loss and I can guarantee you that this is one of the recipes that works best for burning belly fat.

The ingredients are listed below:

- *Cucumbers:*
Cucumbers are low in calories and act as a diuretic. They are also high in dietary in fiber, and water content, which helps flush out fat from the body, keeping the body in an alkaline state.

- *Ginger:*
A study from the Institute for Human Nutrition at Columbia University showed that when participants drank a hot beverage with ginger, they felt fuller and had less chance of overeating. Ginger also creates internal heat that revs your metabolism. A particular study proves that people who include ginger in their diet will lose about 20 per cent more weight than people who don't.

- *Lemons:*
Lemons are high in pectin fiber, which suppresses food cravings and helps the body eliminate waste products by cleansing and detoxifying it. They are also alkaline forming and aid in blasting belly fat.

- *Mint:*
Mint suppresses your appetite and stops cravings. It also soothes the tummy after eating food.

- *Water:*

Water is the essence of life. It keeps your body hydrated, which helps slow down the fat burning process. It also lubricate your joints and muscles during exercise, and helps the blood to supply oxygen to the muscles.

Materials Needed:

- 1 Cucumber
- 2 inch pieces of ginger
- 10 mint leaves
- 1 lemon
- 2 liters of water

Directions:

- Slice all the ingredients and infuse then in water.
- Leave the mixture overnight.
- Drink the liquid content first thing in the morning on an empty stomach Alternatively, juice them all together with a juicing machine.
- Do this daily to get complete relief from belly fat.

Deciding What Foods to Eat:

Our poor lifestyle choices can greatly influence weight gain. Indulge yourself in good eating habits and lifestyle choices.

Below is a check list of things we should bear in mind during our journey to blast belly fat:

- Do not eat any foods that don't grow in nature.
- Do not eat any foods that your great grandmother cannot recognise as food.
- Do not eat any food that you see on TV commercials.

Diet Plan/Guidelines:

• *Avoid Foods That Contain Additives:*

Additives are placed in food to increase their shelve life and to make food more appealing by enhancing their colour, texture or taste. Certain additives, such as aspartame, are made synthetically. Additives simply add no nutritional value to food products, and some can pose a threat to your health.

- ### *Protein Meal Twice a Day:*

There is a saying that goes like this, 'more protein, less fat.' Protein and fats cannot co-exist. If your goal is to lose weight endeavour to consume a protein-rich meal at least twice a day, more preferably for breakfast.

- ### *Consume Low-Calorie Food:*

The trick about weight loss is to consume low-calorie foods and avoid fried foods, which are high in saturated fat.

- ### *Go for Sprouts Than Fatty Snacks :*

Sprouts provides better nutrients than any other snack. They are rich in nutrients and have fewer calories, and when consumed they aid in weight loss.

- ### *Increase Your Consumption of Raw Produce:*

The healthiest foods are those that have been grown organically without the use of insecticides, herbicides or artificial fertilizers. When choosing your fruits and vegetables look for those that are at their peak of ripeness. They usually contain more vitamins and enzymes than the over-ripe or under-ripe. Most fruit and vegetables should be eaten in their entirety, since all their parts contain valuable nutrients. For example, the watermelon. When eating the citrus flesh remove the rinds but eat the white part because it's rich in vitamin C and bioflavonoid content.

- ### *Avoid Over-Cooking Foods:*

Raw food has many advantages over cooked food, but obviously some food can't be eaten raw. When foods are cooked to the point of browning or charring, the organic compound they contain undergoes changes in structure by producing carcinogens. Endeavour to eat your vegetables raw. If that is a big deal for you, feel free to juice them or make a smoothie.

- ### *Use proper Cooking Utensils:*

Although this is in no way related to weight loss, when cooking, it is important to use the right cookware, which includes glass, stainless steel or iron pots and pans. Do not use aluminium cookware or utensils. Aluminium produces a substance that neutralizes the digestive juices leading to acidosis and ulcers. Sometimes the aluminium leaches from the pot into the food. When the food is finally consumed the aluminium is absorbed by the body where it accumulates in the brain and nervous systems, which can eventually lead to Alzheimer's disease.

- ### *Limit Your Use of Salt*

Excess sodium intake can lead to fluid retention in the tissues, which eventually leads to hypertension and can aggravate many medical conditions, including congestive heart failure, certain forms of kidney disease, and premenstrual syndrome. The best way to reduce salt intake is to reduce the amount of junk food you consume, which is high in sodium.

• *Cut the Junk Out*

Try to cut junk food out of your diet. Those foods we can easily grab on the road, such as pizzas, hamburgers, French fries, soda, meat pies, and all forms of processed foods. Artificial sweeteners in these foods can greatly increase your body fat. Instead go for natural and easy snacks such as cashews, almonds, and smoothies. These foods are healthier for your body and immune system.

• *Avoid Carbonized Drinks:*

I know it can be tempting, but avoid any carbonized drink. Instead of carbonized drinks try lime juice, green tea, or tender coconut water.

• *Cut Down On Diet Soda*

You might think that because it's less sweet, it's healthy. Boy, you are making a big mistake! Diet sodas contain artificial sugar to make it less sweet then normal soda. However, it is still unhealthy for you, so cut them out.

• *Keep A Count of Your BMI And BMR:*

It's imperative that you check your Body's Metabolic Index (BMI) and Body Metabolic Rate (BMR) often. Doing this will let you know the amount of calories you should consume, and the amount of calories that are already burnt in your body, giving you better clarity about your body.

• *Drink More Water*

Drink as much water as you can throughout the day. Regular intake of water helps flush out toxins or wastes from the body while keeping it well hydrated. It improves active metabolism and your overall health. Drink at least one 8 oz glass of water or 64 ounces of water per day to get the needed benefits.

• *Reduce Your Sugar Level*

Stick to only natural sources of sugar (Fructose), which are complex carbohydrates. Your body can easily convert complex carbohydrates into sugar, which are beneficial to the body. The bad sugar comes from mostly processed carbohydrates from white breads and other forms of junk..

• *Maintain Your Sugar Level*

A normal fasting (no food for eight hours) blood sugar level is between 70 and 99 mg/dL, while a normal blood sugar level two hours after eating is less than 140 mg/dL. Your sugar level shouldn't go above 140 mg/dl, because your pancreas starts producing more insulin to convert the sugar into fat.

• *Do Not Skip Meals:*

Don't starve yourself because you want to lose weight. Instead, eat a proper balanced diet. Skipping meals will only make your body go into survival mode and start storing the food in the form of fat. It's important you have breakfast, lunch, and dinner daily in your diet. But it's best to have short in between meals rather than three big meals.

• *Increase Intake of Omega 3 Fatty Acids:*

Foods such as salmon and tuna are high in omega-3 fatty acids, which can help you lose belly fat.

• *Increase Intake of Vitamin C:*

Foods such as lemons, oranges, kiwis, and strawberries are rich in vitamin C, which helps to burn abdominal fat, making you look slim, fit and healthy.

• *Eat Fiber Rich Foods:*

Fiber is classified into soluble and insoluble. Soluble fiber dissolves into a gel-like texture, helping your digestion to slow down. This makes you feel full, which greatly helps with weight management. Soluble fiber can be derived from foods such as cucumber, blueberries, beans, and nuts. While Insoluble fiber helps food move through your digestive tract quicker for healthy elimination. Insoluble fiber can be found in foods such as dark green leafy vegetables, green beans, celery, and carrots.

• *Proper Exercise*

Proper exercise is a very important way to lose weight and stay fit. If you can't find time to hit the gym there are various free weight exercises you can do from the comfort of your own home, like the bodyweight squat for your legs, incline push-up for your chest, hip thrust for your abs, walking lunge for your legs, standard push-ups for your chest, and crunch for your abs. All you need is to dedicate a particular time of the day for this, preferably in the morning. Not being able to go to the gym shouldn't be an excuse. You can also go for morning or evening walks or jogs.

With all these said, I know you are getting confused about where to start. Below is a 10 days weight loss plan I created to guide you. Feel free to tweak it to suit your lifestyle.

DAYS	MORNING BEVERAGE	BREAKFAST (WITHIN 9 AM)	LUNCH (WITHIN 1.30 PM)	EVENING BEVERAGE	EVENING INTAKE BY 5	DINNER (WITHIN 9)
Day 1	Water therapy	Oats or protein meal	Small cup of rice + 3 different steamed vegetables (avoid potatoes) + 1 or 2 chapattis	Green tea without sugar	Small cup of sprouts (or) fiber content fruits	Lean protein
Day 2	Water therapy	Protein meal	1 medium cup of wheat rice and veg. salad ddd + char-rchapati + Steamed fchapati + Steamed chapati + Steamed veg or veg salad	Lemon juice & hot water	A cup of veg salad	Lean beef and chicken breast
Day 3	Water therapy	Lean protein meal	2 Sliced Reduced-Calorie Oatmeal Bran Bread	Garlic & Lemon Remedy	A cup of veg salad	A cup of veg salad+2 chapattis
Day 4	Water therapy	Lean protein meal	2 Cups Romaine Lettuce, shredded	Honey and ginger remedy	Nuts like almond	1/2 Cup cooked quinoa

DAYS	MORNING BEVER-AGE	BREAK-FAST (WITHIN 9 AM)	LUNCH (WITHIN 1.30 PM)	EVENING BEVER-AGE	EVENING INTAKE BY 5	DINNER (WITHIN 9)
Day 5	Water therapy	Lean pro-tein meal	1 medium cup of wheat rice and veg. salad chapati + Steamed veg or veg salad	Herbal Cleanse	Boiled potatoes and egg	1/2 Cup Cooked Brown Rice
Day 6	Water therapy	Lean pro-tein meal	1 medium cup of wheat rice + 1 chapati + Steamed veg or veg salad	Lemon, honey and black pepper remedy Leafy greens and salmon	Leafy greens and salmon	1 Cup Steamed Brussels Sprouts
Day 7	Water therapy	Lean pro-tein meal	Small cup of rice + 3 different steamed vegetables (avoid potatoes) + 1 or 2 chapattis	A glass of green juice	Cottage cheese	Beans or legumes
Day 8	Water therapy	Protein meal	Small cup of rice + 3 different steamed vegetables (avoid potatoes) + 1 or 2 chapattis	Green tea without sugar	A cup of veg salad of-nhh sprout	1/2 Cup Cooked Brown rice

DAYS	MORNING BEVERAGE	BREAKFAST (WITHIN 9 AM)	LUNCH (WITHIN 1.30 PM)	EVENING BEVERAGE	EVENING INTAKE BY 5	DINNER (WITHIN 9)
Day 9	Water therapy	Protein meal	Small cup of rice + 3 different steamed vegetables (avoid potatoes) + 1 or 2 chapattis	Lemon juice & hot water	Nuts like almond	Beans or legumes
Day 10	Water therapy	Protein meal	Small cup of rice + 3 different steamed vegetables (avoid potatoes) + 1 or 2 chapattis	Herbal Cleanse	Boiled potatoes and egg eggsprouts (or)A small cup of fiber containing fruit sprouts(or) A small cup of fiber containing fruit	A cup of veg salad+2 chapattis

You mustn't follow this chart completely. It's just for you to get the picture. Feel free to come up with your own chart including the foods that are available to you.

CHAPTER 4

Marvellous Miracles of Honey

I love honey, just as monkeys love bananas. My grand-mother used honey and cinnamon for healing various chronic diseases. One night while we were seated outside attending to numerous patients, I nudged her and she turned to me and asked, "Is there a problem my son?" I asked, "Grandma, why are honey and cinnamon so powerful?" She grinned at me and said, "In Ayurvedic medicine honey is known as Yogavahi, which means, the carrier of the healing values of the herbs to the cells and tissues.

hen combined with cinnamon it reaches the deeper issues in the body more effectively." She also told me that in the olden days honey was referred to as 'the sweet golden liquid,' and was used as a natural cure for many diseases. Now I'll try my best to bring you various honey remedies.

The Honey and Cinnamon Cure

• Heart Disease:

My grandmother died at the grand old age of 98. I believe she owes that to her natural lifestyle. But peculiar about her is that she never visited the hospital. Often my mother offered to take her for check-ups but she bluntly refused. On one particular occasion when she had a grave fall and broke her waist, all effort was made to treat her with the conventional medicine, but she insisted on healing herself the natural way. There is something she did daily to keep heart disease at bay. Every morning at breakfast time she would add honey and cinnamon powder to her bread, instead of the jam everyone else had. This common practice can help prevent heart attack and hypercholesterolemia.

• Arthritis:

I learned this from my grandmother's herbal clinic, where there are usually lots of patients suffering from arthritis. Straight away we apply the paste of honey and cinnamon on the affected area and massage slowly. We also recommend that the patient mix 2 tablespoons of Manuka honey and 1 teaspoon of cinnamon powder into 1 cup of warm green tea and consume this honey cinnamon drink daily in the morning and evening.

Alternatively, some herbalist recommends soaking arthritic joints in hot apple cider vinegar. To do this use a quarter cup of vinegar mix with one half cup of water. You can also soak a cloth into this mixture and wrap it over the affected area.

• Bladder Infections:

If you are suffering from bladder infections my grandmother recommends you mix a teaspoon of cinnamon powder and half a teaspoon of honey in a glass of lukewarm water and drink it. This simple remedy helps destroy the bacteria in the urinary system.

• Toothache:

To remedy severe tooth ache apply a paste of cinnamon powder and honey on the aching tooth.

• Cholesterol:

Nothing lowers cholesterol like honey. By adding a small amount of honey in your daily diet cholesterol levels will be kept in check. The antioxidants in honey helps to prevent cholesterol from being moved out of the blood and into the lining of the blood vessels. To lower your cholesterol level with honey simply add honey and cinnamon powder mixed in boiled water or green tea.

Alternatively, mix one teaspoon of raw honey with two teaspoons of lime or lemon juice in a glass of warm water. Take this first thing in the morning when you wake up.

• Colds:

To banish cold for good, prepare a mixture of honey and a pinch of cinnamon powder in a glass of warm water and drink. This will automatically boost your immune system and help to clear the sinuses.

• Indigestion:

To remedy indigestion, simply sprinkle cinnamon powder on a spoonful of honey. Take this before each meal to relieve acidity and prevent indigestion.

• Hair Loss:

Honey works pretty well in averting hair loss and improving hair growth.

Below are are some effective honey recipes for hair loss:

- Make a paste mixing a tablespoon of honey, a teaspoon of cinnamon powder and olive oil. Apply this paste on your hair and massage thoroughly. Leave it to sit for about 15 minutes and wash off with warm water.
- Grind or juice your onion to get the juice out of it, mix it with a small glass of vodka, and one tablespoon of honey. Massage this mixture on your scalp every night and cover with your shower cap. First thing in the morning shampoo it off and rinse with warm water. A mixture of alcohol and honey stimulates hair growth.
- Another way to use honey for hair growth is to combine ¼ cup of onion juice with one tablespoon of raw honey and then massage the scalp with this mixture every night.
- Lastly, form a mixture of honey and egg yolk and massage onto the scalp. Leave for about ½ hours, then wash off.

• Pimples:

Honey helps with the treatment of oily acne prone skin by feeding the skin with its natural nutrients while killing bacteria that causes acne.

Directions:
Wash the face properly and then apply raw honey to the affected areas. Leave it for about 20 to 30 minutes then rinse off.

Alternatively, apply the honey cinnamon paste on your face and leave it on for about an hour before washing it off with warm water. Repeat this for two weeks for best results.

• Longevity:

Regular intake of tea made with honey and a pinch of cinnamon powder helps strengthen your immune system and protect your body from bacterial attacks.

• Bad Breath:

Baking soda does this for me perfectly fine but honey is another great alternative. Start by mixing honey and cinnamon powder in warm water, and gargle with this mixture to keep your breath fresh.

• Weight Loss:

If your goal is to lose weight, why not substitute your regular table sugar for honey? Refined sugar lacks vital minerals and vitamins. In fact, refined sugar does more harm than good by depleting the body's nutrients, there by impeding the metabolization of cholesterol and fatty acids. This contributes to higher cholesterol and obesity. Drinking a mixture of honey and lemon juice first thing in the morning is an effective anti-cellulite treatment, which helps increase metabolism and prevent obesity.

Below is a simple honey and cinnamon recipe to help you lose weight, lower cholesterol, and regulate blood sugar:

…Cinnamon and Honey Recipe…

I got this recipe from the pages of my grandmother's journal. Below are a few conditions this recipe will help you remedy:
- Improving the body's metabolism and weight reduction
- Lower cholesterol level
- Regulates blood sugar.

Directions:
- Dissolve 1 teaspoon of cinnamon powder in a cup of boiling water.
- Stir it and let it steep for about 20 to 30 minutes.
- Then proceed to filter away the particles.
- Add one teaspoon of honey to it and stir again.

   Take this concoction first thing in the morning on an empty stomach about an hour before breakfast.

• Home Remedy for Cough:

If you are looking for a potent cough remedy then you must be looking for honey. No over the counter prescription can match the powers of honey. Below is a list of the various cough remedies with honey:

Directions:
- Mix an equal amount of honey and lemon grass juice and drink to reduce cough.
- Make your own cough syrup by mixing ¼ teaspoon of cayenne pepper, ¼ ground ginger, 1 tablespoon honey, 1 tablespoon apple cider vinegar, and 2 tablespoons water and drink, and then the cough will soon be gone.
- Another way around this is to boil water with 2 cloves of garlic, 1 tablespoon of oregano, pour it into a cup, add 1 tablespoon of honey, and drink up.

• Honey for Eye Infection:

Believe it or not my dear, honey can be used to counteract eye infection. I first saw this in my grandmother's journal, but was sceptical to prescribe it. Later on I read it in two other trustworthy sources. Due to my curiosity I used myself as a guinea pig and I'm still not blind, even though I had no eye infections. Honey has antibacterial properties, which acts as a humectant, clears eye infections, and provides soothing relief. For this go for raw, unpasteurized honey.

Directions:
- To remedy an eye infection that has spread to the eyelid, mix equal parts of honey and distilled water to make a solution.
- Squeeze two to three drops into your eyes. Apply this two to three times daily until the infection clears.

Alternatively, you can apply oil directly to the eye without any need of dilution. Just place one or two drops of honey directly on the eyes. The honey will collect dirt and discharge, while eliminating it through natural tearing.

• Honey for burn treatment:

When I was 15 years old, we used an aluminium pot to boil water for a bath. Early one morning I went to bring down my boiling pot of water, but the handle was so hot that I could no longer hold on to it, so I dropped it and the boiling water splashed all over my feet. My parents and siblings weren't around to help. Because of my close relationship with my grandmother I knew there had to be a remedy for the burn. I covered up the wound with a wrapper while I tip toed to my grandmother's herbal clinic. She was dazed to see me in such a critical condition. After a thorough examination she told me that I sustained a first degree burn, but there was nothing to panic about. She ran cold water over the burn to cool the affected area to a comfortable level. She then took organic honey and poured about ¼ inch on the affected area, and used her finger to distribute the honey. In less than five minutes the throbbing pain stopped. After leaving the honey on the area for about half an hour and then washing it off, my skin initially felt some numbness, but everything returned to normal within minutes. There was no sign of any burn on my feet. Honey can also be used for burns caused by heat, sun, electricity, cooking oil, and chemicals. For major burns like 3rd degree burns, I suggest you seek medical attention.

• Super food Honey as Natural Insomnia Cure:

My grandmother always advised her sleep-deprived patients to use honey to overcome insomnia. Honey is known to contain sleep amino acid tryptophan that helps overcome insomnia. She also advises that children prone to bed wetting should take one teaspoon of honey before bed, as this is believed to aid water retention and promote relaxation. Honey spikes insulin, which releases serotonin, a neurotransmitter that improves mood and happiness. The body converts serotonin into melatonin, a chemical compound that regulates the length and quality of sleep. Honey is also known to contain omega-3 fatty acids, which research has found reduces fatigue.

• Acid Reflux Remedy with Honey Cider Vinegar Drink:

Acid reflux is usually caused by the excessive production of acid in the stomach. This is caused by the malfunctioning of the lower esophageal sphincter, which allows acid from the stomach to flow backwards into the esophagus by triggering heartburn. Apple cider vinegar aids in digestion by helping the breakdown of fats and prevents acid reflux. It contains acetic acid, which lowers stomach acidity, since the gastric acid produced in the stomach during digestion is full of hydrochloric acid. Honey, on the other hand, has natural antibiotics that coat, protect, and soothe the outer lining of the esophagus. My grandmother used honey and apple cider vinegar as her major remedy for acid reflux. She believes apple cider vinegar helps to destroy harmful bacteria in the digestive tract, and when combined with honey would enhance the healing power of the vinegar.

• Honey Ginger Remedy

I've prepared this remedy a couple of times for my grandmother. It has also being used in ancient times whereby honey is used as a medium for transmitting the benefits of ginger root to the body.

To do this remedy you need:
- 1 tablespoon of honey
- 1 cup of hot water
- 1 tablespoon of freshly grated/finely chopped ginger

Directions:
Put the grated ginger inside a cup and pour hot water. Leave it to steep for about 5-10 minutes then strain the ginger out. Add honey once the drink is cool.

Benefits:
This remedy is suitable for people with digestive issues and it stimulates the body's immunity. It fights toxin and aids in moving food through the stomach and digestive tract. It is also used in the treatment of stomach upset, nausea, vomiting and diarrhea.

Finally, it helps relieve bloating sensation and colic conditions.

Alternatively, you can add fresh lemon juice to increase its effectiveness to soothe scratchy throat, clear sinuses, provide relief for headache, runny nose an cough.

CHAPTER 5

Must Have Natural Remedies for Any First Aid Kit

Whenever I'm going camping or on any vacation, I always pack my First Aid Kit. I remember once I went camping with my girlfriend, and while we were having a good time at the beach, an unknown insect bit her on her thighs.

few minutes later the area was heavily swollen. She went into a panic state, but I continually reassured her that everything was going to be fine. I reached into my first aid box in the trunk of my vehicle and brought out my lavender oil. I used it to soothe the swollen area. In less than 20 minutes the area was completely dissolved and the pain relieved. I believe everyone should have a natural first aid kit as it always comes in handy in emergency situations. Many remedies are multipurpose and can be used for several ailments. I suggest you choose the ones that best suit your needs. I've created a list of recommended first aid items and the cases they can remedy:

Natural First Aid Remedies

Tea Tree Oil:

Tea Tree is one of the most researched essential oils. It is a product of a shrub tree known as Melaleuca Alternifolia, found along streams and swampy areas in its native land of Australia. It's very effective in the cleaning of scratches and abrasions and also in the treatment of fungal infections of the nails, skin, cold sores, and warts. It's also used to reduce itching and swelling resulting from insect bites and calm rashes from plant stings. Tea Tree is very strong and should be diluted before applying to sensitive or irritated skin.

Cuts, Scrapes, and Wounds: Cleanse the affected area with warm water and apply the diluted tea tree oil over the area. Then cover with a bandage if needed.

Insect Bites: Clean the affected area with warm water and dab a little drop of tea tree oil on the bite. This should seize the itching.

Fungal Infections: Dilute tea tree with a little water to reduce its concentration. After, apply the diluted tea tree to the affected area. Repeat this two to four times daily until the infection is completely gone.

Plant Stings: Clean the affected area properly to make sure there is no plant residue left. Then apply the diluted tea tree oil over the irritation.

Tick Removal: Gradually apply a drop of tea tree oil on the tick to loosen its hold. Then gently pull out the tick using a pair of tweezers, after which you disinfect the affected area with diluted tea tree oil.

Lavender Essential Oil:

Lavender is a must have first aid oil. It helps eliminate nervous tension, relive pain, disinfect the scalp and skin, while enhancing blood circulation. Its anti-inflammatory and antiseptic properties can help neutralize venom from snakes and spider bites. The oil is extremely useful in aromatherapy and can blend with many other essential oils. It is very mild and can be applied directly to irritations without dilution.

Burns, Sunburn: Quickly apply lavender essential oil, which helps relieve the pain. After you can apply healing balm, which has arnica, for pain relief.

Sleep Aid: Rub 2-3 drops of lavender oil in your cupped palms, then inhaling draw the scent all the way into your amygdala gland in your brain to calm the mind. Then rub a drop of lavender oil on your palms and smooth on your pillow to help you sleep.

Bruises, Cuts, and Wounds: Drops of lavender oil should be applied to the affected area in order to speed up healing.

Insect Bites: Dab on a drop of lavender to soothe an existing bite, or apply to the skin to deter insects and prevent bites.

Eczema / Dermatitis: Mix several drops of lavender oil with coconut oil and use topically on eczema and dermatitis. I am giving you 100 percent assurance that this works.

Venomous Snake Bite: Wash the affected areas thoroughly with warm water. Try not to move the bitten part, because that will encourage the venom to spread. Apply the oil liberally to the affected area. Seek medical attention immediately.

Nausea or Motion Sickness: To alleviate the symptoms of motion sickness, place a drop of ,lavender oil on the end of your tongue, behind the ears or around the navel.

Black Widow Spider Bite: Lavender essential oil is well known to neutralize the poison from spiders. Apply 5 drops every few minutes until you get medical attention.

Plant Stings: A few drops of lavender oil should be applied immediately after coming in contact with a poisonous plant. Wash the affected areas as soon as possible and apply the oil.

Fainting: To bring a fainted person back to consciousness, sprinkle a few drops of lavender oil on a cloth and hold it towards the victim's nose.

Nervous Tension, Headaches and Migraines: To remedy this situation gently sniff the oil or dab a few drops on your temple to promote calmness and relaxation.

Dandruff: To alleviate dandruff rub several drops of lavender oil into the scalp and massage.

Hay Fever: Are you down with hay fever? Just rub a drop of lavender oil between your palms and inhale deeply.

Nosebleed: To stop a nosebleed, pour a few drops of lavender oil on a tissue and wrap it around a small chip of ice. Push the tissue covered ice chip up under the middle of the top lip to the base of the nose and hold for as long as comfortable or until the bleeding stops.

Cold sores: To remedy this put a drop of lavender oil on a cold sore.

Clove Oil

Clove oil has antimicrobial, antifungal, antiseptic, antiviral, aphrodisiac, and stimulating properties. The oil is widely used for the treatment of various health disorder, including toothaches, cough, indigestion, asthma, headache, stress, and blood impurities. The most common use of clove oil is for dental care. It can also be used on the skin to numb bodily pain.

Numbing: Clove oil should be diluted with another essential oil, before use. It acts as an effective pain killer when applied topically. It's great for injuries that need time to heal.

Toothache: Clove oil can be used to numb your gums, mouth and teeth during a toothache. It should be applied on the gums or teeth to reduce dental pain and further prevent infections.

Aloe Vera Gel

Aloe Vera has been applied to the skin to treat wounds, skin infections, burns, and many other skin conditions. The dried latex is usually taken as a laxative. Aloe vera also helps in the treatments of inflammatory skin conditions, genital herpes, dandruff, and for numerous other conditions.

Burns and Sunburn: This plant is great for soothing sunburns and other minor burns. To remedy sunburn clean the area with water and apply aloe vera on the affected areas. You can also add a few drops of lavender oil to boost the healing effect.

Heat Rash: Aloe vera gel should be applied gently on affected areas to calm the itching.

Witch Hazel

Witch hazel has a mild astringent and is mainly used for bruises, sores, and swelling. It is also widely used to prevent infection, repair broken skin, and to stop minor bleeding. The major component of the extract include tannin, gallic acid, catechins, proanthocyanins, flavonoids, essential oil, choline, saponins and bitters. It's also used to dilute essential oils for topical applications.

Spot and blemish control: Witch hazel helps reduce the inflammation on a pimple. Drop a few drops of witch hazel on cotton wool and dab on the affected area. Daily use of witch hazel can also help in cases of acne.

Soothe and heal diaper rash: To heal your baby from rashes, drop a few drops of witch hazel on cotton wool and dab on the affected areas. You will see improvements immediately.

Sunburn: Application of witch hazel to sunburn skin helps speed up the healing and prevents peeling and flaking of the skin.

Shrink bags under the eyes: Application of witch hazel helps tighten up loose skin and reduce the bagginess.

Swelling : To reduce the swollen area soak a clean piece of cotton wool on witch hazel solution and gently dab it on swollen areas.

Cuts and scrapes: Soak your cotton wool with a few drops of witch hazel and dab it on the affected areas to help cleanse the area and prevent it from infection while encouraging the wound to heal faster.

Soothe and reduce external haemorrhoids: Mix witch hazel with aloe and apply on external haemorrhoids. The bleeding and itching will be reduced significantly. Blisters: To dry unbroken blisters apply witch hazel solution to the affected areas and fasten with adhesive bandage.

Varicose vein relief: Soak a white cloth in witch hazel and lay it on your legs. This helps to reduce pain and swelling from varicose veins. The witch hazel helps to tighten the veins, relieving the discomfort temporarily.

Bruises: Apply to the area 3 times a day to speed the healing time of the bruise.

Treat chicken pox blisters: To treat chicken pox mix together 1 tablespoon of honey, 15 drops of lemon essential oil, 40 drops of lavender oil, 5 drops of peppermint essential oil, 1 teaspoon of carrot seed oil, and 1/2 cup Aloe Vera gel. Mix thoroughly and add 1/2 cup distilled witch hazel. Pour the mixture into a spray bottle and use on affected areas, avoiding the eyes.

Plant stings: Wash the affected areas thoroughly and apply white hazel to reduce itching and relieve swelling.

Insect bites: Soak a clean cloth with white hazel and dab on affected areas to reduce itching and swelling.

Tick removal: Sprinkle a few drops of witch hazel to help loosen its hold. Grasp the tick with tweezers and pull firmly. After removal, disinfect the area by dabbing the skin with witch hazel.

Bach Rescue Remedy

Rescue Remedy is a combination of five of the original Bach Flower Remedies, which are especially beneficial when you find yourself in traumatic situations, such as after getting bad news, stress, emotional upset, before an exam or job interview, emergencies, or all kind of situations where you suddenly lose balance mentally. The remedy quickly gets you back in your normal balance so that you can calmly deal with any situation at hand. This remedy can also help children relax at night or calm them during tantrums. Rescue Remedy is safe for anyone to use and it does not have any negative side effects.

Shock, Accidents, Trauma, Stress or Emotional Distress: For tense situations like these pour a few drops of the Bach Rescue Remedy under the tongue and hold it for a few minutes before swallowing. You can also mix the drop in a small glass of water and gradually sip it. For an unconscious person place the drops on their lips. For pets, place the drops in their drinking water.

Arnica Oil

Arnica oil is found to have antimicrobial and anti-inflammatory properties, and may be helpful for treating or relieving muscle aches, spasms, pulled muscles, or rheumatic pain. Arnica oil is a must have oil to place in your first aid box. Arnica belongs to clan of flowering perennial plant from the daisy family. Native to Europe and Siberia, it also grows in North America, especially in mountainous regions. Arnica is a remedy of choice for trauma and muscle injury. It also comes in homeo-pathic pellets and drops for internal use and is mostly used for relieving headaches, trauma, and shock. Avoid using the gel, cream or salve on broken skin. When using the pellets, hold under the tongue until it's completely dissolved.

Swelling: When used as a topical treatment, arnica helps brings down swelling by stimulating fluid movement around the area, thereby flushing out water and other liquids that contribute to the puffiness. Arnica also helps stimulate white blood cell movements and promotes healing. Because of this, arnica helps get rid of bruising quicker too.

Hair loss: A diluted form applied to your scalp can help increase local blood circu-lation, thereby promoting hair growth.

Bruising, Swelling, Sore Muscles, Sprains, and Strains: Rub the topical arnica on the affected area and massage thoroughly to alleviate discomfort and speed the healing process.

Headaches: For headaches take 4 pellet or drops of Arnica.

Trauma or Shock: For trauma or shock of an accident administer 5 pellets or drops of Arnica 30 times.

Calendula Cream:

 Calendula can be found in creams, oils, and ointments. It's traditionally used for abdominal cramps and constipation. Calendula has anti-bacterial, anti-fungal, anti-inflammatory, astringent, and wound-healing properties. When applied topi-cally it reduces skin inflammation and irritations.

Skin dryness or chapping: Calendula oil is a great moisturizer for dry skin and for severely chapped or split skin. It soothes the area and reduces the pain. Apply the oil to the affected areas and massage thoroughly.

Inflammation: Calendula has anti-inflammatory properties, which helps lessen swelling from injuries. It is also great in the treatment of sprained muscles or bruis-es and helps treat spider veins, varicose veins, leg ulcers, and chilblains. Apply a little quantity to affected areas and massage thoroughly.

Baby care: The oil helps relieve diaper rashes, which can extremely irritate an infant. Apply a little quantity around the affected areas and massage properly.

Minor cuts and wounds: The antiseptic and antimicrobial action of the oil help speed up healing of wounds and minor cuts, and also benefit insect bites, acne, and bed sores. After cleaning the affected area, apply calendula cream.

Skin issues: Calendula oil can be used in the treatment of eczema, psoriasis, dermatitis, and other skin problems. Clean the infected surface and apply a little portion of the oil then massage thoroughly. Calendula oil's antifungal action is also great for treating athlete's foot, ringworm, and jock itch.

Blisters: If a blister has broken apply calendula to speed healing and prevent infection.

Sunburn: Cool the affected area and apply calendula to soothe the burn and promote healing.

Insect Bites and stings: Rub a little calendula cream onto the bite to soothe itching and irritation.

Rashes: Clean the area properly and apply calendula to the affected area as often as needed to reduce irritation.

Sea Buckthorn Oil

Sea buckhorn contains unique high fatty acid content and a wealth of other nutrients, which makes it one of the most health-promoting herbal oils. The oil is a natural anti-inflammatory, antiviral and high in antioxidants. The anti-inflammatory properties promote wound healing and the formation of healthy tissues. When applied topically it can give the skin temporary orange colour due to the oil's high carotenoid content, which normally fades as the oil is absorbed into the skin.

Sunburn: Cool the affected areas and apply sea buckthorn oil to soothe the skin and lessen the pain associated with sunburn.

Minor Burns and Scalds: Cool the burn with a soak cold water towel, then apply sea buckthorn oil to reduce the pain and heal the burn.

Cuts, Scrapes, and Wounds: Pour a few drops to the wound and gently massage the infected area to accelerate healing and reduce scarring

Relieves dry eyes. Oral supplementation of sea buckthorn oil in individuals with dry eyes for at least three months.

Cayenne

Cayenne has been used for a variety of ailments, including heartburn, delirium, tremors, gout, paralysis, fever, dyspepsia, flatulence, sore throat, atonic dyspepsia, haemorrhoids, menorrhagia in women, nausea, tonsillitis, scarlet fever, and diphtheria. And most of all, it has shown remarkable results in the heart attack cases. It is said that the cayenne must be of high potency (at least 90,000 heat units) to stop a heart attack. If heart attack is your major concern, it is worth travelling with cayenne on your trips. Cayenne powder comes in capsules or tincture.

Minor Bleeding: For quick cessation of bleeding apply a bit of cayenne powder topically over the wound.

Heart Attack: Add a teaspoon of ground cayenne to a cup of warm water and administer it to the victim. If the victim is unconscious and may not be able to drink the mixture, use cayenne tincture or extract and put a few drops underneath their tongue.

Ginger

If you are prone to motion sickness or digestive upset, ginger is the best thing to have in your natural first aid box. It has a special way of easing a queasy stomach due to motion sickness, and it also helps relieve discomfort associated with indigestion or gas and bloating. Ginger is packaged in various forms (capsule, powder, essential oil, crystallized or fresh). Choose the form that best suits you.

Nausea or Motion Sickness: Place a few drops on a neat towel and inhale until the symptom subsides. Alternatively, you can chew slices of fresh ginger root or take it in powder or capsule form every 15 minutes until nausea subsides. If you think you might vomit the ginger, if swallowed, hold the ginger in your mouth and gradually suck it. For motion sickness take 3-4 grams of ginger in capsule or powder form 45 minutes before departing.

Indigestion, Gas or Bloating: To remedy this, dilute ginger essential oil in a carrier oil and gently massage over your upper abdomen. Alternatively, chew on crystallized ginger or fresh ginger root, or sip a tea made from ginger root.

Goldenseal

Goldenseal is a strong anti-septic, anti-fungal. It is also a good anti-bacterial for the skin when applied topically. It's very potent in the treatment of diarrhea caused by bacteria. It's excellent as a sore throat gargle and any upper respiratory or sinus problem where there is yellow mucous. Goldenseal should be taken at the first sign of respiratory problems like colds, or flu, and to prevent further symptoms from developing. It is also used to reduce fevers and relieve congestion and excess mucous. Goldenseal can be used topically as an antiseptic and to stop minor bleeding. Goldenseal may also help with allergic rhinitis, hay fever, laryngitis, hepatitis, cystitis, and alcoholic liver disease. Goldenseal cleanses and promotes healthy glandular functions by increasing bile flow and digestive enzymes, therefore regulating healthy liver and spleen functions. It is available in capsule, powder, and tincture. Goldenseal should not be taken more than 10 days in a row. Pregnant and breast-feeding mums should avoid goldenseal.

Wounds: Goldenseal is a great organic and pain-free solution to clean and promote healing for certain wounds. It also comes in a capsule form, which can be opened and sprinkled directly into the wound, then bandaged. This will help speed the healing process up.

Food Poisoning or Traveler's Diarrhea: Take 1,000 – 1,500mg of goldenseal immediately and repeat the same dosage three times a day until symptoms are gone

Cold or Cough: Take 1000mg at the first sign of cold, cough or flu. Repeat this dosage till symptom clears.

Oil of Oregano

Oregano oil is produced from the perennial herb oregano and it's rich in antioxidants. Oregano oil offers immense health benefits and is known as one of the most potent natural remedies in existence. It acts as an immune stimulant and kills bacteria, virus, fungus, and parasites. It is also widely used as a remedy for traveller's diarrhea, and the common cold. Taking a few drops of oil in juice or water may also provide some relief from a sore throat.

Because of its strong nature it should be evenly diluted with a carrier oil (olive, coconut, sunflower, etc.) To avoid skin irritation Oregano should not be taken internally for more than two to three weeks continuously.

Food Poisoning and Traveller's Diarrhea: Take 3-6 drops of oregano immediately after noticing any symptom of food poisoning. Repeat the dosage three times daily until the symptom subsides.

Digestive Issues: For digestive issues take 3-6 drops two to three times a day to help relieve intestinal gas and digestive problems.

Cough and Cold: 3 -6 drops should be taken at the first sign of a cold. Then it should be repeated threee times per day before meals for at least five to ten days. For cases of coughs and bronchitis take for the duration of illness to mobilize mucous and ease spasticity of the lungs.

Injuries, Aches and Pains: Sprinkle 3 drops of oregano on the affected areas and massage properly to decrease inflammation and ease pain.

Headaches and Migraines: Pour a few drops on your finger and massage onto your temples and between your eyebrows. Repeat this process as needed and be careful not to get any into your eyes.

Toothaches and Mouth Sores: Mix a few drops of oregano with some drops of carrier oil and swish it in your mouth for a few minutes. Spit it out when finished. Repeat as needed.
Fungal Infections: Apply diluted oregano on fungus infections such as athlete's foot, and toenail fungus.

Insect Bites: Apply a drop of diluted oregano oil to ease itching from mosquito and ant bites.

Tick Removal: Apply a few drops of oregano to the area where the tick is attached to loosen its hold or use tweezers to remove the tick.

Venomous Bites and Stings: Clean the surrounding and apply diluted oregano liberally. Oregano oil will help to neutralize venomous bites from snakes, spiders, scorpions, and bees while waiting for necessary medical attention.

Neem

Neem are well used to soothe skin irritations and to support oral hygiene. They are also used as a natural insect repellent. The capsules are used internally to purify the body, and offer benefits that parallel the actions of bitters, tea tree, garlic, and aloe. A diluted solution can be used for cuts, burns, boils, and blisters.

Cuts: Carefully wash cuts and wounds with diluted solution of neen, as an antiseptic, to protect from infections, help stop bleeding, and promote healing.
Burns: Wash with a diluted solution to cool burns and give antiseptic healing. It has remarkable healing effects.

Boils: When used topically it helps heal boils, removing pus and germs quickly without leaving any marks.

Blisters and Rashes: Sponge with diluted solution on tender skin and itching skin for relief.

Oral gargle with Neem for dental care: Take ¾ cup warm water and mix with ½ tsp Neem. Gargle the mixture, and repeat this twice daily to protect against infection and oral ulcer.

For pimples and acne: Wash face daily three to four times with diluted solution of Neem aid. Alternatively, you can also mix a few drops with your facial cream and apply on pimples. Check for allergy to Neem before using.

Anti-dandruff / Head lice / Scalp diseases: Make a solution of Neem aid with ½ cup of water and 2 tsp neem aid , apply on head/scalp and hair , gently rub for few minutes. Leave for two hours, and then wash off.

Neem bath for chickenpox to assist healing and leave no marks: Mix 20-25 ml of Neem aid to one bucket of water. Use the water to take your bath.

As a sponging to bring down high fever: Take a bowl of water (about 1 litre), mixed with 3 tsp of Neem aid, then Sponge head with this solution for ½ to 1 hour as required.

Use it as a mosquito and insect repellent: Mix 25 ml of Neem aid with 50 ml sesame oil. Store the mixture in a bottle. Apply on body as required to protect against mosquito bites. Do the same if you are outdoor to prevent leech and insects.

Licorice tea:

Licorice tea is naturally sweet and mainly used to soothe sore throats. It also helps aid smooth digestion. Licorice tea is also useful in extreme cases of constipation.

Probiotic for Diarrhea:

Diarrhea is a condition in which faeces are discharged from the bowels frequently and in a liquid form. Probiotic products have special microorganisms like bacteria or yeast in them, which are believed to reach the bowel, where they help fight the germs causing the diarrhea. So always remember to bring probiotics along with you each time you travel a far distance

Vitamin D for Flu:

Flu is a respiratory illness caused by a virus. It is highly contagious and usually spread by the coughs and sneezes of an infected person. Numerous studies about the flu have shown that people who have lower levels of vitamin D are more likely to get flu. If you are coming down with flu, it's best to take vitamin D in doses of 50,000 units a day for three days to treat the infection

Hydrogen Peroxide for Colds and Flu:

Administer a few drops of 3 percent hydrogen peroxide (H_2O_2) into each ear. You will hear some bubbling, but don't panic, as this is completely normal and you will possibly feel a slight stinging sensation. Wait until the bubbling and stinging subside (usually 5 to 10 minutes), and then drain it with a tissue or cotton wool. Repeat the same process for the other ear. This remedy has recorded remarkable success in the treatment of cold and flu

Ginger for Nausea:

This remedy is pretty simple. All you need to remedy nausea is to dice up a piece of ginger and swallow it. Ginger also has anti-inflammatory properties and helps ward off bacteria and fungi.

Pure Water for Hiccups:

To remedy hiccups, tell a friend to hold down the tragus of your ear, in order to close your ear canal while you drink a full cup of water. This remedy always

CHAPTER 6

Marvellous Miracles of Apple Cider Vinegar

I got to know about the numerous uses of Apple Cider Vinegar (ACV) when I was 10 years old. My mother and grandmother used it for a lot of different things ranging from cooking, health purposes, cleaning, garden care, hygiene, and many more.

M y grandmother also used it in most of her natural remedies. My grandmother told me that ACV has been used as a medicine for centuries, and since 400BC, Hippocrates, the father of modern medicine, and others, have used vinegar and vinegar mixed with honey as an energizing tonic and a healing elixir. Apple Cider Vinegar is made by crushing apples and squeezing out the liquid. Bacteria and yeast are added to the liquid to start the alcoholic fermentation process, and the sugars are turned into alcohol. In a second fermentation process, the alcohol is converted into vinegar by acetic acid-forming bacteria (acetobacter). This action leaves it rich in bioactive components such as acetic acid, gallic acid, catechin, epicatechin, caffeic acid, and more, giving it potent antioxidant, antimicrobial, and many other beneficial properties.

• Remove Dandruff

If you are still battling dandruff, apple cider vinegar is one of the best remedies to ward off dandruff. Most women spend a fortune battling dandruff without the knowledge that the true remedy for dandruff is sitting on their kitchen shelf. The solution is simple. Just mix equal parts of apple cider vinegar and water in a spray bottle and spray onto your hair after shampoo. Leave it for 15 minutes before rinsing it off. Repeat this process at least twice weekly and your dandruff will go away. This is due to the acidity in dandruff, which makes it hard for fungus that contributes to the growth of dandruff in the hair.

• Soothe A Sore Throat

This is my go-to remedy for a sore throat. I have given up on over the counter medications, now I simply rely on my remedies. To soothe a sore throat simply mix one tablespoon of apple cider vinegar, one teaspoon cayenne pepper, and three teaspoons of organic honey in a glass of warm water and drink. I'm yet to find any cough syrup as potent as this. I have recommended this remedy to countless people and they all come back with positive feedback. The capsaicin in the cayenne paper helps to alleviate pain while the apple cider vinegar and honey have antibacterial properties.

• Diabetes

My grandmother recommends this remedy for most type 2 diabetic patients. The acetic acid present in vinegar lowers blood sugar by preventing the compete digestion of complex carbohydrates. This is accomplished by increasing the uptake of glucose by bodily tissues i.e. vinegar slows the absorption of carbohydrate into the blood, or slows the breakdown of starches into sugars. Studies have found that taking vinegar at bedtime lowers blood sugar levels in people living with type 2 diabetes by up to 6 percent by the morning. Another study found that vinegar treatment helped improve insulin sensitivity in 19 percent of people living with type 2 diabetes, and 34 percent of those with pre-diabetes.

The question may arise, if vinegar was that effective, why then aren't doctors prescribing it? I guess it's because vinegar is so cheap and there's no profit to be draw funding for large studies. If you want to control any type of diabetes, consume vinegar before meals and at bedtime.

• Heart Health

Apple cider vinegar plays a huge role in heart health. It contains an antioxidant known as chlorogenic acid, which has been shown to inhibit oxidation of LDL cholesterol and improve your overall health by preventing cardiovascular diseases. A particular study conducted on rats shows that apple cider vinegar lowered their cholesterol, while another study on rats lowered their blood pressure with apple cider vinegar.

• Skin Irritation

Apple cider vinegar is a good remedy to have in your natural first aid kit. It works for a variety of skin inflammations, from bug bites to poison ivy to sunburn. All you need to do is apply it directly to the irritated area.

• Warts

Warts are those small, hard, benign growths on the skin, caused by a virus. The high level of acetic acid present in apple cider vinegar helps remedy warts. To do this, apply cider vinegar to a cotton swab, rub over the affected area, and leave it overnight

• Energy Boost

Looking to boost your overall energy level? Then why not try apple cider vinegar? It contains potassium and enzymes, which helps banish fatigue, and its amino helps prevent lactic acid build up in your body.

• Repel Fleas On Your Pets

I use this for my dog all the time and I can testify to its effectiveness. Combine equal parts of apple cider vinegar and water, pour into a spray can. and spray on your dog's fur saturating the entire coat. Do this daily until there is no sign of fleas.

• Reduce Heartburn

It might sound a little bit counterintuitive to treat stomach acid with acid vinegar, but several studies suggest that apple cider vinegar works by correcting low acid, and hence reducing heartburn. Simply take 1 teaspoon of apple cider vinegar followed by a glass of water.

• Balance Your Digestive System

Apple cider vinegar stimulates digestive juices that helps your body to breakdown food. Also, taking a tablespoon of apple cider vinegar with water before meal can help to reduce gas.

• Sinus Congestion

Apple cider vinegar is one of the well-known remedies for sinus congestion that works. It helps to break up and reduce mucous in your body, which helps to clear your sinuses.

• Helps Get Rid of Candida

Candida is a genus of yeast and is the most common cause of fungal infections. Apple cider vinegar is very effective in getting rid of candida yeasts. It is rich in natural enzymes that can regulate the presence of candida in the body and helps encourage the growth of healthy bacteria, which in turn minimizes the overgrowth of candida. To cure candida, simple take 2 tablespoons of apple cider vinegar with a glass of water daily.

• Clear Up Your Skin

The best beauty products aren't that expensive and apple cider vinegar is certainly one of them. It helps absorb excess oil and reduce fine lines. For smooth and supple skin apply a washcloth soaked in diluted apple cider vinegar to your face. Its protective acidic layer will make your skin glossy and supple. This works by restoring the proper pH levels of your skin, and beta-carotene helps to counter future skin damage. Also, to reduce pimples, acne, or age spots on the face, dab diluted apple cider vinegar on and leave it overnight.

• Oral Health

To get rid of mouth odour and whiten your teeth, gargle with a cup of diluted apple cider vinegar. It's very important to dilute with water before swallowing, because apple cider vinegar is very acidic. Putting it undiluted directly into your mouth can damage the tissues of your mouth and throat.

• Deodorant

Apple cider vinegar is an effective deodorant, more reliable than most store bought ones. It kills the odor causing bacteria. Simply dab a little under your arms for a refreshing start to the day.

• For Hair

Apple cider vinegar is great for your hair. It helps boost hair shine by closing the hair cuticles, and it also removes unwanted product build up from your hair. Regular use of apple cider vinegar will help revive your hair, leaving it soft and supple. Directions: After shampooing, pour the apple cider vinegar and water into a spray bottle and spray onto your hair. Let it sit for a few minutes before rinsing with warm water. The use of a conditioner afterwards is not needed, because the ACV will leave your hair feeling smooth and soft.

• Age Spots

To fade age spots within two weeks, begin by applying a mixture of 2 teaspoons of apple cider vinegar and 1 teaspoon of onion juice on the darkened area of the skin. My granny uses this remedy a lot. Try it and see for yourself!

• Asthma

Appl cider vinegar works fairly well with asthma, as its acidity helps hydrochloric acid perform its job, which explains why apple cider vinegar relieves acid reflux and asthma. This remedy is one my granny recommends for asthma patients. Directions: Dilute one tablespoon of apple cider vinegar in a glass of water and drink it in sips over about half an hour. If the wheezing idos not subside, repeat the process. If you are still not relieved of your symptoms soak a cotton pad into appl cider vinegar and hold it against the insides of your wrist, while applying adequate pressure.

• Arthritis

For patients with arthritis, my granny always advises that they should mix 2 egg whites, ½ cup (125 ml) apple cider vinegar, and ¼ cup (60 ml) olive oil, and massage this concoction on the sore joint. Also they can take a glass of diluted apple cider vinegar before a meal.

• Athlete's Foot

Athlete's foot is a common infection of the webs of the toes and soles of the feet. When caused by fungus it may spread to the palms, groin, and body. One of the remedies in my granny's journal involves soaking your feet twice a day in an equal part of apple cider vinegar and water. Apple cider vinegar can be applied on the affected areas several times a day and before bedtime.

• Nose Bleeding

To stop nose bleeding, have the victim lay his head back and then soak a cotton ball in apple cider vinegar and place it in the bleeding nostril. This should help stop the bleeding

• Blood Pressure

To lower your blood pressure, prepare a mixture of 1 tablespoon of honey and apple cider vinegar in a glass of water. Drink this concoction twice daily. Doing this helps balance out the sodium levels in the body due to the high potassium values in both substances. Apple cider vinegar and honey also contains magnesium, a mineral that helps relax blood vessel walls thereby lowering high blood pressure.

• Bone Health

Apple cider vinegar is rich in minerals such as manganese, magnesium, phosphorus, calcium, and silicon. These minerals help to sustain bone mass and fight osteoporosis. Start by taking apple cider vinegar diluted with water, and boost it with needed diets and minerals.

• Bruises

To treat bruises dissolve 1 teaspoon of salt in ½ cup of warm apple cider vinegar and apply it to the bruise as a compress.

• Burns

Apple cider vinegar helps to balance the skin's pH factor, its acid/alkaline balance. As with all parts of the body, when there is chemical balance, healing is supported. To heal any kind of burn, apply apple cider vinegar to the burn area. Doing this will help reduce the pain, disinfect, and supply nutrients required for healing. For large sunburn areas prepare a vinegar bath by adding two cups of apple cider vinegar to a bathtub of warm water and soak in it for about 15 minutes. Also note that your skin will not burn on contact with vinegar, unless there's an open wound, which is not common with cases of burn. You will only feel a tingling sensation without pain.

• Colds

Apple cider vinegar helps to alkalize the body, and when the body is in an alkaline state it becomes more effective at fighting viruses responsible for common cold and flu. My granny recommends drinking 1 tablespoon of apple cider vinegar diluted in half a cup of water several times a day. If you have a chest cold, there is a particular remedy in my granny's journal that calls for soaking a piece of brown paper in vinegar, then sprinkling one side of it with black pepper. Place the peppered side of the paper on your chest, then cover with a towel and leave for about 20 minutes.

• Constipation

Being constipated means your bowel movements are difficult or happen less often than normal. This can happen for various reasons like a change in your usual diet, eating a lot of dairy products, irritable bowel syndrome, not enough water and fiber, or taking antacid medicine containing calcium or aluminium. There is no need to panic, because it happens to everyone from time to time. To remedy this naturally my granny suggests eating more fruits and vegetables and taking a daily tonic of diluted apple cider vinegar (2 or 3 teaspoons to 8 ounce of water).

• Diarrhea

Apple cider vinegar is a natural remedy for diarrhea. This is due to pectin, a water soluble fibre in apple cider vinegar, which helps absorb water into the intestine and bulk up the stools. Also, the high pectin concentration in the vinegar soothes the irritated lining of the colon. To remedy diarrhea mix 2 tablespoons of apple cider vinegar into an 8oz glass of water and drink three times daily.

• Ear Infections

Apple cider vinegar changes the pH of the ear canal thereby creating an environment where bacteria and viruses cannot thrive, according to Dr Robert O. Young and Shelley Redford Young, in their book, The pH Miracle.

Heat the vinegar and test on the inside of your wrist for the temperature. Place a few drops in the painful ear and cover with a piece of cotton. Lie with the painful ear facing up to allow the vinegar to penetrate.

• Eczema

Eczema is a chronic skin disorder identified by skin inflammation of the epidermis, which results in rashes and skin scaling on different parts of the body. Vinegar contains lactic, acetic, and malic acids containing antibacterial and anti-fungal properties, which combat dry skin and skin infections, relieving inflammation, itchiness, and dryness. To help relieve the itching and dryness of eczema, apply a 50/50 mixture of apple cider vinegar and water to the affected areas.

• Menstrual Problems

To reduce the flow of a heavy period take a diluted glass of apple cider vinegar (3 teaspoons to 8 ounces of water) first thing in the morning.

• Leg Cramp

To help stop painful muscle cramp take 3 tablespoons of apple cider vinegar mixed with 8 ounces of water. Doing this helps the body absorb calcium and magnesium, which helps protect against painful leg cramps.

• Morning Sickness

A pregnant friend of mine told me that she stopped experiencing the usual nausea and vomiting in the morning after she started drinking a glass of diluted apple cider vinegar. I recommended this remedy to a few more people and they all had positive results with it.

• Sore Muscles

To remedy sore muscles, mix 1 tablespoon of apple cider vingar with cayenne pepper. With the aid of a towel apply this to the sore muscle for about 5 minutes, and reapply if the need arises. If you feel the soreness all over your body have a vinegar bath by adding 2 to 3 cups of vinegar into your bathtub filled with warm water .

• Fabric Softener

I do this a lot. To soften your clothes, add 1/3 cup of white vinegar to your laundry before the final rinse cycle. (Please only do this during the final rinse cycle as the water is filling, or already full. If you add it to your spin cycle – this might bleach your clothes and make it smell like vinegar.) As an alternative, you can add 1/2 cup of white vinegar to the fabric softener dispenser in the washing machine before starting a laundry cycle instead. Doing this keeps the clothes neat and odourless.

• Clean Your Washing Machine

This method also calls for baking soda. All you need to do is run a normal wash cycle (on hot) and place ½ baking soda and 2 cups of white vinegar in the machine, once it's filled with water. Doing this breaks down the dirt particles and keeps the hoses nice and clean.

• Hiccups

Hiccups are an involuntary spasm of the diaphragm and respiratory organs, with a sudden closure of the glottis and a characteristic gulping sound (that's the dictionary definition). To stop this, simply sip a glass of diluted apple cider vinegar, which will stop your hiccups at once.

• Insect Bites and Stings

To soothe insect bites, like mosquitoes, bee and wasp stings, apply undiluted apple cider vinegar to the affected area.

• Boil Eggs

While boiling eggs, adding vinegar prevents the breaking of the shells.

• Ulcers

To remedy aan ulcer, I strongly suggest you use a cold-pressed vinegar made from organic apples. This ensures you are getting an ample supply of vitamins, minerals, and enzymes with each serving. Take 2 teaspoons of diluted apple cider vinegar daily. Apple cider vinegar can also be added to hot tea or sprinkled on to salads and mixed with honey.

• Urinary Tract Infections

To maintain the right pH balance in your urinary tract drink a daily tonic of diluted apple cider vinegar. When the urinary tract has the right pH value, it keeps bacteria and yeast infections at bay. Another alternative is to drink a juice of 2 teaspoons of apple cider vinegar and cranberry. Cranberry juice is a well-known remedy for urinary infections because it prevents bacteria from attaching to the walls of the urinary tract.

• Varicose Veins

Apple cider vinegar is a well-known remedy for varicose veins. Start by soaking a cheesecloth into apple cider vinegar. Then tie the bandage around your thighs or lower legs. Leave the bandage on for about half an hour. Remove the bandage and wash your legs. Alternatively, apply it directly to your legs early in the morning and in the evening, and massage thoroughly. Before commencing this remedy, try it on a small part of your leg to see whether your skin is sensitive to it first.

• Shingles

To remedy itching and shingles rashes, take a bath of warm water mixed with 1 cup of apple cider vinegar. Alternatively you can apply undiluted apple cider vinegar directly to the rash.

• Corn and Callus Treatment

For corn and callus treatment, start by soaking the affected areas in apple cider vinegar, diluted in warm water. Follow this by rubbing the area briskly with a coarse towel, and then use a clean pumice stone to rub the affected areas, then apply apple cider vinegar and cover it with a bandage overnight. In the morning prepare a fresh apple cider vinegar soaked bandage for daytime use.

• Flatulence

Soaking beans in apple cider vinegar prior to cooking, helps minimize gassing.

• Night Sweats and Hot Flashes

For menopausal women apple cider vinegar helps to eliminate hot flashes and night sweats. Start by taking diluted apple cider vinegar tonic morning and night.

• Clean Barbecue Grill

To clean your barbecue grill, spray a solution of apple cider vinegar and water on warm grill. Leave it for about ten minutes. With the aid of a scouring pad soaked in the vinegar, scrub grill, as the dirt will loosen easily.

• Yeast Infection

Apple cider vinegar is known to be one of the strongest antibiotics ever. It kills viruses and helps restore the vagina's pH level while preventing yeast fungi from thriving and infecting the vagina with further yeast infection. It helps to re-colonize the intestines and vagina with a friendly bacteria, which acts as a powerful guard to stop the bad bacteria (candida) from returning. Simply soak a clean cloth or cotton ball in diluted apple cider vinegar for two to three minutes. Place the cloth on the walls of your vagina or around your penis. Repeat regularly until the yeast infection is gone. Alternatively, you can mix a glass of apple cider vinegar in a glass of herbal tea or filtered water and drink regularly two to three times daily on an empty stomach to prevent yeast infection.

• Sinus

Apple cider vinegar is a well known remedy for sinuses. It contains vitamins B1, B2, A and E, Calcium, Potassium, and Magnesium. These vitamins help to clear sinus cavities and reduce allergy symptoms. When taken orally it helps break up mucus and clear the airways. To treat sinuses sip a glass of diluted apple cider vinegar throughout the day. Alternatively add ½ - 1 tablespoon of organic apple cider vinegar to a cup of warm filtered water, and stir properly. Wash your palms properly, pour some of the mixture into it, and snort it up one nostril at a time, while using the other hand to plug the free nostril. Repeat on the other side too.
Also, you can mix equal amounts of apple cider vinegar and water together. Heat the mixture for a few minutes then turn off the heat and inhale the steam by closing your mouth and eyes. Keep inhaling for a few more minutes to relive sinus infection.

• Weight Loss

Although there is no medical proof for this, a research published in the Journal of Functional Foods show that participants who drank a tablespoon of apple cider vinegar mixed with 8 ounces of water prior to eating had lower blood glucose levels compared to participants who didn't. It's generally believed that apple cider vinegar also acts as an appetite suppressant and increases your body's metabolic rate, by reducing water retention. Acetic acid, which is the main component in vinegar, is said to interfere with the body's ability to digest starch, and this starch-blocking power can help you shed few pounds. Dr. Jarvis recommends you take 1 to 2 teaspoons of apple cider vinegar plus 1 glass of water before meals three times a day.

CHAPTER 7

Marvellous Miracles of Aloe Vera

I can still remember sitting side by side with my Grandma, as she told me beautiful stories about her younger self. She told me how beautiful she was as a young girl and how several men asked for her hand in marriage. One of the reason she choose Grandpa wasn't because he was a known wrestler, but because he had the heart of a child, even with his fierce look. Grandma's stories are the type you ould love to listen to all day long. Most of the knowledge I have as an adult was transferred to me by my Grandmother. Often, I worked next to her in her herbal centre and I did most of the errands for her. Part of the full time duty assigned to me was to plant and cater for the aloe vera plants.

Grandma gave me a list of patients under her therapy whom I should deliver the aloe vera or aloe vera water to. My job was to make sure the aloe vera was delivered at the right time to the right people. I did this for some time and that landed me the name "Aloe Vera Boy" by my peers. You wouldn't believe it if I tell you that the common aloe vera that grows in your backyard holds immense health benefits and uses. Below is a simple method I use to whip up aloe vera water:

...Powerful Aloe Water Recipe...

You will need:
- Aloe plant leaf (or 2 tablespoons of edible aloe vera gel)
- Knife
- Spoon
- Blender
- 1 cup of water.

Direction:
- Start by cutting out a leaf from the aloe vera plant.
- Slice the leaf open with a sharp knife (down from the middle).
- Gently scoop out the gel, and be sure to avoid colleting the yellow part of the plant, which is located below the rind.
- Mix 2 tablespoons of aloe vera gel with one cup of water in a blender.
- Blend until it's smooth.
- Store the juice in an air-tight container.
- Your aloe vera water is now ready.
- Aloe vera water can be used to treat constipation and heartburn.
- It detoxifies your bowels while reducing fecal yeast and improving gastrointestinal function.
- It can also be used in the treatment of inflammatory bowel disease.

• Aloe Vera for Facial Scrub

Aloe Vera works well as a skin exfoliate. Exfoliating your skin helps reduce the appearance of blemishes and blackheads. It's recommended that you exfoliate your skin at least three times a week to wash away dirt and oil from your skin. To make your own aloe vera facial mask mix 1 tablespoon of baking soda to 2 teaspoons of aloe vera to make a paste. Apply the scrub on a clean face and massage in a circular motion. Be watchful not to get it too close to your eyes because that will hurt greatly. When you have covered a greater portion of your face, let it sit for a few minutes. Rinse and moisturize using virgin coconut oil. Alternatively, you can combine ¼ cup of brown sugar, 1 tablespoon extra-virgin oil and 1 tablespoon of aloe vera gel. Mix and apply on your face. Massage in a circular motion. Rinse off the scrub by alternating between cold and warm water.

• Treat Burns

Aloe Vera gel is one of the best remedies for burns. I know this for sure because my Grandmother used it extensively to treat patients with burns. I am the guy who plants all the aloe vera used in my Grandmother's herbal centre. She does this by splitting the leaf length wise into two halves and scraping out the gel inside. She will then apply the gel directly to the burn. The gel will soak into the skin, immediately soothing and relieving the patient. Aloe vera can also be used on sunburn, thermal burns, and areas of any sort of skin irritation or inflammation.

• Treat Scalds

A scald is caused by hot liquid being spilt on the skin. Aloe vera helps cool and soothe the skin, while its antibacterial properties will help stop further infections. It penetrates deep into your skin to rebuild skin from the lowest level. In my own experience applying aloe vera to scalds, healing occurred 50% - 75% faster than conventional treatment. To create a homemade burn healer mix aloe vera gel and vitamin E oil into a jar and apply to the affected area.

• Soothe Insect Bites, Stings and Itching

Histamines are the cause of an adverse reaction to insect bites, stings from mosquitoes, biting flies, scorpions, and bees. Histamines rise to the surface of the skin to battle toxins left in your skin from the saliva or stinger that penetrates into the surrounding dermal layers. The itching and redness associated can be alleviated with aloe vera gel. Just split open the aloe vera and massage the gel onto the affected areas. A good alternative I recommend is to apply aloe vera to the skin in a liquid form. To do this simply make an aloe vera spray by blending equal amounts of aloe vera leaves and water. Add the resulting mixture into a spray bottle and spray on the affected area several times a day for instant relief.

- ## Prevent Permanent Tissue Damage From Frostbite With Aloe

Frostbite is injury on the body caused by exposure to extreme cold, which affects mostly the nose, fingers, feet or toes, resulting in gangrene. When you expose your skin to the extreme cold for a prolonged period of time, your cells begins to draw oxygen away from the extremities and carry the blood to vital organs, which is constricted and dilates blood vessels in spurts. Aloe is used to treat frostbite because it has been proven to increase the blood flow to the affected areas. Doing this allows the restricted vessels the opportunity to expand and repair, while simultaneously reducing pain, redness, swelling, and inflammation. To treat frostbite apply aloe gel directly to the affected area twice daily. I advise that you don't seize treatment until the frostbite has healed completely.

- ## Aloe for Rashes and Allergic Reactions

I once had a mysterious rash. I spoke with a friend and she advised me to put aloe vera on it. I tried it out and to my surprise it cleared up within two days. Rashes can be caused by a number of factors, such as eczema, hives, poison ivy or heat rashes, which are often accompanied by severe pain and discomfort, itching, and swelling. To remedy this skin condition, clean the affected area and apply aloe. It all comes down to the severity of your rashes. For rashes covering wide areas, triple the dosage by applying aloe gel three times daily.

- ## Help Heal Herpes Outbreaks

Herpes are a group of virus diseases caused by herpesviruses, affecting the skin (often with blisters) or the nervous system. Aloe vera helps to activate the process of self-healing, whereby the body's own immune offers the best course of treatment. Aloe hsa also shown to be effective against a variety of viruses, including influenza, herpes, and HIV. When taken orally, it helps boost your immune system to fight against viral infection. It can also help reduce the occurrence of viral symptoms.

- ## Fight Athlete's Foot

Athlete's foot is a fungal infection that begins between the toes. It occurs mostly in people whose feet have become very sweaty while confined within tight fitting shoes. The area becomes red, flaky, and blistering, which is usually swollen, burning, painful, and itchy. Some people might say that its counterintuitive to use a oe for Athlete's foot since it thrives on damp places, and how can a plant that keeps your skin wet help to reduce or prevent a fungus that is usually treated by drying the affected area? Aloe vera is capable of this because it contains protein called 14 kDa that prevents the fungus from spreading. To treat Athlete's foot with aloe vera, mix aloe vera with tea tree oil to create an ointment. Apply on the affected area at least twice a day until the infection subsides. Alternatively, you can mix four ounces of aloe vera gel with a teaspoon of tea tree oil in a spray bottle and spray on the affected area twice daily. Make sure you dry your feet before applying.

• Prevent Pimples and Treat Acne

Aloe vera is a natural astringent that helps remove excess oil, dirt, and dead skin cells, which clog the pores and cause bacterial infections. It purifies your blood and stimulated cell growth, while healing damaged and scarred skin. It is anti-inflammatory, which helps reduce the redness, inflammation, and pain associated with acne. The hormones known as gibberellins and polysaccharides present in aloe vera help to kill acne-causing bacteria. To use aloe vera to remedy acne, extract the gel from fresh aloe and apply it on affected area. Let it sit for about 5 minutes before rinsing off. Then moisturize the area (coconut oil is my personal favourite) Repeat this twice daily for best results. Another alternative is aloe vera and lemon. Start by blending a reasonable amount of aloe vera and lemon and apply the paste to the affected area before going to bed. Leave it overnight. Upon waking up in the morning rinse it off your face. Repeat this regularly for best results. Aloe vera can also be mixed with turmeric and honey with a few drops of rose water to make an excellent paste for acne. Repeat the same process as above.

• Soothe Psoriasis with Aloe Vera

Psoriasis is a skin disease marked by red, itchy, scaly patches. Aloe vera is known to be very effective in minimizing psoriasis severity when compared to steroid creams. Its anti-inflammatory properties help to soothe inflamed and irritated skin, while reducing redness and swelling. Aloe gel is a powerhouse of essential antioxidants and vitamins, which help fight psoriasis, and repair and restore damaged skin cells. When taken orally it flushes out toxins from the body, boosts the immune system, and fights psoriasis. For psoriasis aloe vera juice should be drank on an empty stomach first thing in the morning. You can blend it with a non-citrus fruit to make it a bit tastier. Alternatively, you can blend aloe vera with calendula leaves in a blender, and apply the paste on the infected skin three to five times daily. Leave the paste overnight for faster results. Aloe vera can also be mixed with baking soda to reduce the intensity of itching caused by psoriasis. Mix aloe vera gel with baking soda in a 2:1 ratio. Apply the paste and leave for 10 minutes. Wash off with clean water. Baking soda can be replaced with Epsom salt. The essential minerals of Epsom salt enhances the healing process of infected skin, soothes flare-ups, and reduces swelling in psoriasis.

• Prevent Scarring and Stretch Marks

Aloe vera plays a huge role in getting rid of stretch marks, as it has approximately 5 nutrients, 18 amino acids, 20 minerals, 200 enzymes, and 12 vitamins, such as Vitamin A, B1, B2, B12, C, E, etc, which play a huge role in the treatment of stretch marks and helps to make your skin glow. Aloe vera's anti-inflammatory properties help to heal stretch marks, it doesn't only clear stretch marks, it also prevents future occurrence. When applied regularly it helps regenerate and rejuvenate the skin, which in turn removes stretch marks on the skin. Aloe vera is capable of penetrating deep into the skin, while nourishing the skin and repairing it from the damage caused due to stretch marks. The antioxidant present in aloe vera helps repair the damaged skin cells and enhances the generation of new skin cells to replace stretch marks. To remedy stretch marks, rub aloe gel directly on the stretch marks, let it dry, and then rinse it off your skin with lukewarm water. You can also mix aloe vera with vitamin A and E oil. Apply it onto the stretch marks, leave it for a few minute, then wash off with warm water. Another alternative is to mix aloe vera with lemon or lime juice and repeat the same process outlined above. I advise you to apply any of the above remedies at least once a day until the stretch marks have disappeared.

• Help Get Rid of Rosacea

Rosacea is a condition in which certain facial blood vessels enlarge, giving the cheeks and nose a flushed appearance. People who suffer from rosacea usually have bloodshot and itchy/irritated eyes also, known as ocular rosacea. Some experience tightness or thickness of the skin, raised patches, and even swelling. Aloe vera is a miracle treatment option for rosacea and applying aloe vera topically increases the moisture while rejuvenating your skin to reduce the redness and irritation associated with rosacea. To remedy rosacea, wash your face properly and apply aloe gel to the affected areas. You might begin to feel tightness and a burning sensation, but there is no need to panic, as it is expected. After ten minutes, the redness should begin to subside. After about a week of continuous usage, you should begin to see a significant improvement in your condition.

• Shrink Warts

Warts are small, hard, benign growths on the skin, caused by a virus. To treat, gently rub the aloe pulp on the wart. Do this daily for an extended period of time. You can leave some aloe pulp on the wart, just remember to cover it with gauze.

• Reduce Wrinkles and Rejuvenate with Aloe

Aloe vera helps remove dead skin cells from the skin. Doing this helps improve the skin's texture and diminishes the appearance of wrinkles. One thing I have observed from using aloe vera is that my skin became smoother and supple. It might also interest you to know that aloe vera contains over 200 nutrients and active ingredient, which helps nourish and improve the overall health of your skin. Collagen is a part of the connective tissue in the skin that helps in firmness, suppleness, and constant renewal of skin cells. Fibroblast is a cell in connective tissue which produces collagen. As a person ages their skin produces less Fibrobast, which leads to lesser collagen, and may lead to wrinkles, saggy skin, and an aged appearance. Aloe vera helps the skin produce more collagen, which rids the skin of wrinkles. Aloe also helps to lock in moisture and replenish the skin.

• Help Eliminate Eczema

Aloe vera works well in the treatment of eczema. A friend of mine had eczema and he called me asking for the remedy. He believed in me when it comes to natural remedies and thought I was the expert in that niche. I recommended aloe vera to him hoping that it worked. One week later he called to inform me that the rash had reduced by 50%. I told him to try taking aloe vera juice orally. He started drinking 6 ounces daily coupled with a healthy diet, and within 7 days he got me a new cell phone in appreciation for curing his eczema. Eczema is a condition which requires both inside and outside cures. Several studies conducted on this issue have shown that the plant has the ability to give a bolstering effect to the immune system and help heal epithelial tissues.

• Encourage Hair Growth: Clean Out Your Hair Pores with Aloe

Most times the pile-up of grease and dirt can accumulate in your scalp's pores resulting to blockage of the pores, which may result in suffocation and inflammation of the hair follicles, and the chances of developing an infection increases. The good news is that aloe vera can help get rid of all the dirt in your pores, allowing fresh hair to push through and grow easier, while preventing infection or inflammation.

• Aloe For Your Exfoliating Experiments

By now you should have known that exfoliating the skin reduces the appearance of blemishes and blackheads. It recommended that the skin be exfoliated at least three times a week to wash away dirt and oil, and revive your skin. Exfoliating scrubs away the first layer of oil and dead skin cells on your face, and aloe vera does wonders in that department. Personally I've tried a few, which am going to list below:

• Soothing Aloe Vera and Baking Soda Scrub

Start by mixing 1 teaspoon of baking soda with aloe vera gel. Apply the mixture on your face and massage thoroughly. Make sure you wash your face before applying the scrub. Be careful not to get it close to your eyes. When you are done scrubbing, wash it off your face with a mild soap and moisturize. My favourite moisturizer is coconut oil.

• Homemade Olive Oil, Aloe, and Sugar Scrub

This scrub penetrates deeply to exfoliate. Soothe, smooth, feed, nourish, and hydrate the skin. To prepare this scrub mix ¼ cup of brown sugar, 1 tablespoon extra virgin oil, and 1 tablespoon of aloe vera. Apply the mixture on your skin and gently massage in a circular motion. When you are done, rinse the mixture alternatively with cold and warm water. Pat dry skin and moisturize.

• Reduce Hair Dandruff

Aloe is anti-fungal, which when used regularly will help get rid of dandruff. Aloe vera should be rubbed on the scalp and left overnight. Upon waking up in the morning wash out with warm water and a mild shampoo containing aloe vera and rinse with cold water. Repeat this for five days. At the end of the fifth day, you should begin to see noticeable changes. Your scalp should be less dry and flaky. Alternatively you can mix aloe vera juice with coconut milk and wheat germ. Apply the mixture to your hair and massage thoroughly. Wash and rinse off with aloe vera shampoo afterwards.

• Replace Aloe with Conditioner for Silkier, Smoother hair

Aloe vera can also be used as a hair conditioner. In fact, it's one of the best conditioners known. The gel is rich in keratin, which is a protein found naturally in hair cells, and it's easily absorbed into the scalp. It contains about 20 amino acids, which gives it more power to strengthen your dry hair. Using aloe vera as a hair conditioner, will give you sleek and shiny hair. To use aloe vera as a conditioner apply the gel directly on your hair, starting from your scalp and working your way down. When you are done with the massage wrap your hair in a towel or cover hair with a shower cap. Let it sit for about 15 minutes before washing off.

• Makeup Remover

Aloe vera is the best alternative to oil based makeup remover. For what it's worth you know exactly what you are putting on your face. Refrigerated aloe vera gel soaked in cotton balls also provides a great compress for tired, puffy eyes.

• Treat Minor Vaginal Irritations

Aloe vera has being proven to clear up candidiasis and prevent recurrences due to its anti-fungal properties. Vaginal infections can be treated by applying aloe vera externally and by aloe vera juice. It recommended you take four to six ounces of aloe vera daily to help treat vaginal irritations.

• Drink Aloe Vera Juice to Relieve Gastrointestinal Disorders Like Indigestion

Drinking aloe vera juice can help in various digestive problems, such as acid reflux, stomach bloating, flatulence, and irritable bowel syndrome. It does this by cleansing the gastrointestinal tract, reducing colonic build-up and promoting normal transit of waste matter through the bowel. This is possible because of the laxative compounds barbaloin, aloin, and aloe-emodin present in aloe vera. Aloe vera also has an anti-inflammatory effect on the lining of the GI tract.

• For Rheumatoid Arthritis Pain

Arthritis is a chronic progressive disease causing inflammation in the joints and resulting in painful deformity and immobility, especially in the fingers, wrists, feet, and ankles. A study published in the Journal of the American Podiatric Medical Association in 1994 reported that aloe vera reduced the inflammation in joints affected by arthritis. It also supports the autoimmune reaction when the body attacks its own tissue, as happens with rheumatoid arthritis. Aloe vera can be used directly on the joints or you can drink aloe vera juice to help decrease inflammation

• Alleviate Asthma

There are many factors that can trigger an asthma attack, some of which are dust mites, certain types of grass, pollen, or strong emotional reactions, especially stress. Inflammation is the leading cause of pain and also the primary cause of asthma since it causes the interior of the airways to swell, making it difficult for air to pass through. Aloe vera is anti-inflammatory and so it makes perfect sense to use it to alleviate asthma. You can do this by boiling leaves in a pan of water and breathe in the vapor to alleviate asthma.

- ## Drink to Lower Blood Sugar Levels—Especially for Diabetics.

Research has shown that the intake of aloe vera juice can help improve glucose, and can therefore be useful in the treatment of people with diabetes. It decreases swelling and encourages faster healing of wounds in patients with type 2 diabetes. Take a tablespoonful of aloe juice twice daily to help regularize insulin flow and lower blood glucose levels naturally, and open constricted blood vessels to facilitate the delivery of oxygen and nutrients to your bloodstream, and also to combat the vascular disease that can accompany diabetes. Apply pure aloe vera gel to diabetic boils to reduce inflammation and irritation. Apply pure aloe vera gel to minor cuts and scrapes to soothe them and promote healing.

- ## Aloe Vera For Bad Breath

Aloe vera can be used as a remedy for halitosis. Personally I believe it's a safer alternative than commercial products, as at least you know what you are taking in. Due to its anti-fungal and antibacterial properties it helps kill bacteria as well as help fight tooth decay. It also helps boost the body's ability to create collagen, which helps strengthen your weak and swollen gums. To use aloe vera in this fashion, simply dissolve ¼ cup of aloe vera in ½ cups of apple juice. Drink the mixture to soothe acid indigestion, which is the primary cause of bad breath.

- ## Aloe As A Sore Throat Remedy

Sore throats are often caused by virus or allergy. Aloe vera, when taken regularly, can help bolster the immune system to help ward off sore throats. It cleanses and detoxifies the digestive system while lowering the acidity of the gastric juices found in the stomach that are responsible for sore throats. To soothe sore throats, gargling with an aloe vera solution can give you immediate relief and boost your overall health. To make a basic gargle for sore throat get ¼ cup witch hazel extract, 1 teaspoon vegetable glycerine, 1 tablespoon apple cider vinegar, and ¼ cup aloe vera gel. Mix all ingredients up and gargle as desired.

- ## Aloe Vera for Receding Gums

Aloe vera is anti-inflammatory which makes it very effective in reducing the inflammation of gums and to activate cells that are important for tissue repair. Its anti-bacterial properties help keep the infection away from your mouth. To use aloe vera for receding gums, every morning and night when you have brushed and flossed put some aloe vera gel on your brush and brush your teeth once again with it, then wash your mouth. Alternatively, aloe vera can be used as a mouth wash. After brushing your teeth in the morning add some water to aloe gel and mix thoroughly to form a thick consistency. Gargle with the mixture for a while and spit out. Do this every time your brush your teeth.

• Aloe for Acid Reflux Relief

If you've ever felt a burning sensation moving up into your chest after having a meal, then you might have had acid reflux disease. Next time this happens there's no need to panic. Aloe vera is a natural alternative to get rid of heartburn. Simply drink 2 or 3 ounces of aloe vera juice. This will help soothe the irritated internal skin.

• A Natural Treatment For Conjunctivitis

Conjunctivitis is the medical term for pink eyes. It is contagious and can be often caused by bacteria or viruses. Aloe vera is anti-bacterial, antifungal, and antiviral, which makes it perfect for the treatment of pink eye. To treat pink eye infection with aloe vera, simply place a few drops into each eye two to three times daily. I advise that you continue this treatment for a few days more, after the symptoms have disappeared. Doing this will help prevent the infection from recurring.

• Get Rid of Contusion

Contusion is a region of injured tissue in which blood capillaries have been ruptured. Aloe vera helps soothe the skin and clear up the discoloration caused by contusion. When applied topically on the skin, it pumps moisture into the skin, which helps speed up blood vessel repair, so the contusion disappears faster. To remedy contusion, start by cleaning the affected area with water and gentle soap. Then break the aloe vera leaf to get out the gel. Apply aloe vera gel topically to the contusion. Repeat this several times daily until contusion heals.

• Aloe Vera For Constipation

Are you constipated? Why not try aloe vera juice? Aloe vera contains a chemical called chloride, which is potent and an effective stimulant laxative. Its fluid is drawn into your stool, making it softer to ease your bowl movement. You should also know that aloe laxatives can interfere with the absorption of prescription drugs, and taking aloe juice for more than two consecutive weeks can result in loss of electrolytes, especially potassium. Women who are pregnant and menustrating should avoid aloe juice.

• Aloe Vera For Heat Rash

Heat rash occurs when your skin isn't exposed to circulating air, and sweat is accumulated at the surface. It sinks down, clogging your glands. Babies are typically affected by this, more often in their diaper region or around the folds of the neck. Also hot weather and sweaty exercise can lead to heat rash. Aloe vera gel can be applied topically on the rash to soothe it.

• Aloe For A Healthier Heart

High cholesterol occurs when the level of cholesterol becomes elevated and leads to fat build up in the arteries. This build up can lead to heart disease, heart attack, and strokes. Lucky enough, high cholesterol and triglyceride levels can be lowered naturally with aloe vera. Taking reference from a medical study, aloe vera gel is administered to patients with heart disease and high cholesterol. When a patient was given 100mg of Aloe Vera for a period of three months, the result confirmed that aloe vera gel decreased cases of heart attack, strokes, and chest pain. This result was due to the anti-oxidant and dietary property of the aloe vera plant that causes the reduction of high cholesterol.

CHAPTER 8

Amazing Uses of Hydrogen Peroxide

I never knew that hydrogen peroxide held such immense benefits. I always see the topic on the web but I thought it was just another internet myth.

Then one faithful night I had sinus issues and had no alternative cure. It was so severe that I had to do something before I could get a good night's sleep, so I called a very good friend who is a huge remedy enthusiast. He suggested that I add 3% hydrogen peroxide to 1 cup of chlorinated water and use it as a nasal spray. My immediate response was, "Hell no," and he said, "Not like you have a choice, bro" and hang up the phone immediately. Initially, I couldn't bring myself to do it, but I had to be free from my sinus issues, so I tried it and it worked. Hydrogen peroxide (H_2O_2) is the only germicidal agent composed only of water and oxygen. Its oxidizing properties allow it to react with bacteria, viruses, spores, and yeasts, making it a great disinfectant. Hydrogen peroxide is considered the world's safest all natural effective sanitizer.

• Get rid of acne and boils

If you are battling with acne, I strongly suggest you try hydrogen peroxide. It helps kill the bacteria which caused the acne while cleansing the area. To do this apply it directly on the infected areas, only once. Do not overdo this, as otherwise you could kill the good bacteria.

• Replace Chlorine

Adding chlorine in pools can be unpleasant and irritating for many. Hydrogen peroxide is a better and non-toxic alternative.

• Cure Canker Sores

This remedy is as old as the hills. It's the first go-to remedy for canker sores. Hydrogen peroxide is antibacterial and antiseptic. It kills the bacteria in and around the mouth, healing canker sores and reducing inflammation. Start by gargling diluted hydrogen peroxide (mix with water) in your mouth for around two minutes and spit out.

• Bad Breath

If you can't get rid to bad breath and regular toothpaste isn't working for you try hydrogen peroxide. Start by gargling with a diluted glass of hydrogen peroxide. For a more potent combo, make a paste of baking soda and hydrogen peroxide and brush your teeth and tongue with it. This will completely eradicate bacteria from your mouth and help whiten your teeth.

• Fight Food Fungus

A friend of mine told me about this, and she swore it worked for her. Personally, I haven't tried it, but so many people testified that it cured their foot fungus infections. Start by mixing 3% hydrogen peroxide to one gallon of clean lukewarm water. Then soak your feet for about 30 minutes, rinse off, and pat dry. Do this every morning and night.

• Treat Cold / Flu

Boy, this one works well. I know because I've tried it. Start by administering a few drops of 3% hydrogen peroxide into each infected ear. It starts working within 2 to

3 minutes in killing flu or colds. You will experience a bubbling and in some cases a mild stinging. Wait until the bubbling and stinging subsides, then roll over, and drain the H202 onto a tissue, and repeat on the other ear. Repeat this process two or more times at one or two hour's intervals, until no bubbling occurs.

• Get Rid of Ear infections and Clear Out Ear Wax

To get rid of ear infections, simply use the hydrogen peroxide by putting a few drops into ear. This is just for mild ear infections. For severe ones I suggest you see the doctor. You can also use hydrogen peroxide to clear up excessive wax in your ear. Start by adding a few drops of olive oil, followed by hydrogen peroxide. Then keep your head tilted for about a minute then tilt it back the other way to let the mixture drain out.

• Sinus Infections

Many have testified to the effectiveness of this remedy. Personally I haven't tried it before but a friend of mine walked me through the process. It goes like this: put 1 tablespoon of 3% hydrogen peroxide into a spray bottle of your choice, and add 1 tablespoon of water into the bottle. Keep the mixture 50-50, which will make a 1.5% formula. Spray this into your nose and blow it back out, as this will kill your sinus infection.

• Tackle Toothache

I remember on one particular occasion when I had an awful toothache, my granny instructed I put some diluted hydrogen peroxide in my mouth and hold it there for about 10 minutes. To my surprise it worked. But as with everything in life, moderation is the key.

• Take A Detoxifying Bath

Whenever I'm ill, I simply take a detoxifying bath to clean all the germs away frim my body. I do this by adding two quarts of hydrogen peroxide into my bathwater and soak for about half an hour.

• Yeast Infections

Hydrogen peroxide produces a natural bacteria in the vagina while killing yeast. Start by mixing 1 teaspoon of 3% hydrogen peroxide with 1 cup of water. Use this mixture to rinse the vagina once a day until symptoms disappear.

- # Deodorant

I ditched my deodorant a long time ago for baking soda, which happens to work best for me. But recently I found out that adding Hydrogen peroxide to this mix is way more effective. Every morning after my hot shower. I put a few drops of hydrogen peroxide on it and wipe my under arms. This helps to clean the area and gets the underarm ready to hold the baking soda. I then add a few sprinkles of baking soda on another cotton swab and use it to wipe under my arm while spreading the baking soda for a good coverage. This shouldn't make a paste, but rather seem like dusting.

- # Clean Your Contact Lenses

My sister uses contact lenses and one way she get rids of build-ups is with hydrogen peroxide. If you are quiet and observant you will notice that hydrogen peroxide is the active ingredient in every lens cleaner, and it does the job pretty well.

- # Tile and Grout Scrub

Cleaning dirty floors is a chore I dread, and since I'm the kind of guy that always looks for the easy way out, I use of hydrogen peroxide. Sometimes I mix it with baking soda as this helps deep clean and disinfect the floor. It's especially useful for grout, which can be extremely difficult to scrub.

- # Whiten Your Nails

This is one of the remedies I learnt from my sisters. To whiten your nails soak a reasonable amount of hydrogen peroxide into a cotton ball and dab it onto your nails.

- # Laundry Bleach

The harsh fumes from chlorine are dangerous to inhale and can sometimes lead to severe respiratory issues over time. The chemical residue also remains on your clothes, which can sometimes cause harsh irritation. That's why I prefer using hydrogen peroxide, which happens to be a non-chlorine bleach. Start by adding ½ cup of hydrogen peroxide alongside with your regular laundry detergent.

- # Fruit and Veggie Sanitizer

In the absence of vinegar I use hydrogen peroxide to sanitize my produce before juicing them. Simply spray a food-grade hydrogen peroxide on your fruits and vegetables. Let it sit for few minutes before rinsing off, then pat dry. Using hydrogen peroxide helps kill harmful organisms in your produce.

• Odor Eliminator

I own a cat and a dog and sometimes these pets can cause severe odor around the house. To eliminate odor I simply apply baking soda and hydrogen peroxide to the problem areas. Let it sit for a while then wipe clean.

• Lighten Your Hair

You can also use hydrogen peroxide to lighten your hair over time. To do this simply mix equal amounts of hydrogen peroxide and water. Add this mixture into a spray bottle and spray it on your hair. Comb hair afterward for an even distribution. When done regularly the hair will start to show blonde highlights. This method of hair lightener gives you total control of how light you want to go, and it's not harsh on hair.

• Disinfect Your Toothbrushes

To disinfect your toothbrushes against bacteria, simply pour some hydrogen peroxide over them. I do this regularly to keep my toothbrush free from germs.

• Soften Calluses and Corns

To soften calluses and corns on feet, simply mix hydrogen peroxide and water in a bowl and soak your feet.

• Disinfect Small Wounds

One of the well-known uses of hydrogen peroxide is disinfecting small wounds. It's a natural antiseptic and widely used to clean wounds to prevent infection.

• Help Heal Boils

To heal boils simply pour half of a bottle (8 ounces) of hydrogen peroxide into warm bath water and soak.

• Disinfect Your Countertops

This is my mum's favourite way to disinfect countertops. She does this by mixing equal parts of hydrogen peroxide and water, then sshe epours the mixture into a spray bottle. Using the spray bottle she sprays directly on the surfaces, then wipes clean.

• Clean Your Mirrors

Recently I discovered that hydrogen peroxide leaves no streak on my mirrors, unlike other commercial cleaners I have used. I use it mostly to clean my bathroom mirrors and it's quite effective in getting rid of dirt and germs that have accumulated on the mirror over time. I do this by simply spraying it on, then wiping clean.

• Wash Out Your Toilet Bowl

To disinfect your toilet bowl, pour a reasonable amount around the bowl, let it soak for about 30 minutes, then scrub and rinse out. When you're done douse the toilet brush with hydrogen peroxide, as this will disinfect the brush and keep it clean.

• Remove Tub Scum

There is nothing I dread more than the ring that builds up around my bath tub. But I've found a way to get rid of this scum. Pour hydrogen peroxide into a spray bottle and spray on the soap scum, dirt, and stains in your bathtub. Let it sit for at least 30 minutes. This loosens the grime making cleaning easier.

• To Clean Grout / Tiles

Another name for my mum is Mrs. Clean, as she always wants the whole place sparking clean. I learnt this way of cleaning tiles from her. Start by making a paste of hydrogen peroxide by mixing it with flour. Apply the paste on tiles and cover it with plastic wrap. Let it sit overnight, then the following morning rinse it off, while cleaning the ties. Alternatively, to clean grout, mix baking soda with hydrogen peroxide. This helps lift the stains as well as disinfecting for a deep clean. Your tiles and grout will come out looking bright and sparkling.

• Kill Mold

Vinegar works well in this department, but I've found that you can also use hydrogen peroxide to achieve the same result. Apply hydrogen peroxide anywhere you find mold in your house and wipe clean. This will help clean and detoxify the area

• Canine Emetic

If your dog consumes foods that are toxic, simple administer hydrogen peroxide, as this will cause the dog to throw up. This simple remedy can save a dog's life if done quickly.

• Bloodstain Remover

To remove blood stains from textiles, simply dab the stained areas with hydrogen peroxide and rinse with cool water before you commence washing. Doing this will naturally pull the stain out leaving the fabric soft and clean. Please note that hydrogen peroxide can bleach fabric, so before commencing it pays to try it out on areas that aren't visible before treating the problem area.

• Keep Salad Fresh

Have you ever wished that your vibrant plate of salad can stay fresh for longer? Well, I'm glad to tell you that there's a way to accomplish this. Start by prepare a mixture of half cup of water and a tablespoon of hydrogen peroxide (make sure to use food grade) then spray the mixture over your salad.

• Vegetable Soak

Using hydrogen peroxide as a vegetable soak helps to kill bacteria and neutralize chemicals. Start by adding ¼ cup of 3% H_2O_2 to a full sink of cold water. Then soak the vegetables for about 20 minutes, clean, and pat dry before putting them in the refrigerator. Doing this will prolong the freshness of your vegetables. If you have time constraints, spray your vegetables with a solution of 3% hydrogen peroxide. Let them stand for a few minutes, then rinse and pat dry.

• Get Rid of Stubborn Caked On Foods

Still having trouble getting rid of stubborn caked on food on your pots and pans? Worry no more, as I've got the perfect solution for you. Make a paste of hydrogen peroxide and baking soda, and rub the paste on those difficult areas. Let it sit for a few minutes before scrubbing it away with warm water. The baking soda acts as an abrasive, while the hydrogen peroxide helps break up the particulates.

CHAPTER 9

Marvellous Miracles of Coconut Oil

Coconut oil is phenomenal and miraculous. It's the most important thing in my home. I use it for virtually everything. I usually buy coconut oil in bulk and stock thee jars in the store, so I don't run out. I can't overemphasis the importance of this oil. I really don't know what my life will be like without it.

This chapter outlines all the amazing uses of coconut oil I know of. I'm sure after reading this, you will get obsessed with the oil yourself.

• Weight Loss

Coconut oil and weight loss…what's the connection between the two? Coconut oil will help you lose weight when you substitute it with other unhealthy oils used in cooking. It contains saturated fat, which doesn't get packed away as fat easily, rather it's sent straight to the liver to be metabolized, which in turn boosts your energy level. It also helps suppress your appetite. Whenever you have unnecessary cravings just take two tablespoons of coconut oil.

• Prevent Stretch Marks

Coconut oil is great at nourishing damaged skin. Although there is no proven way of totally preventing stretch marks, because most of the times it's widely a genetic issue. Coconut oil is rich in vitamin E and fatty acids, which penetrates deep down in the skin to provide and retain moisture in the skin. I suggest you apply it 1 to 2 times daily throughout the course of pregnancy.

• Cold Sores

Virgin coconut oil has proven to be an effective natural remedy for treating cold sores (oral herpes) as it is both antiviral and antibacterial. Cold sores are inflamed blisters in or near the mouth, caused by infection with the herpes simplex virus. Cold sores spread from person to person by close contact, such as kissing. Coconut oil contains coconut fat and lauric acid, a fatty acid that the body transforms into monolaurin. Monolaurin prevents the virus from spreading. Apply coconut oil directly to the sore several times a day.

• Energy

Coconut oil has no cholesterol. The medium chain fatty acids present in coconut oil are broken down and used for energy. They produce energy, not fat. Also you have to know that medium chain fatty acids do not have a negative effect on blood cholesterol and it helps protect against heart disease.

• Yeast Infections

Coconut oil contains a full spectrum of antifungal, antiviral, and antibacterial properties. And also substances like lauric acid and caprylic acid, which help fight yeast. The medium chain fatty acids penetrate the cell membrane and weaken the cell, so it disintegrates. Then white blood cells go in and gobble up the waste material, while killing the yeast, virus, and bacteria.

• Moisturize Your Skin

Coconut oil is well known for its moisturizing property. It delivers a refreshing burst of moisture, which penetrates the skin and truly heals it. Using coconut oil can make your body feel oily, to avoid this, make sure you take the needed amount of time (at least 15 minutes) to massage the oil thoroughly on your body.

• Conditioner

Coconut oil makes a perfect deep conditioning hair treatment. It helps condition, strengthen, and repair hair. Take a generous amount of coconut oil and massage it onto your hair. Rinse it out after ten minutes. A small amount can be rubbed into dry hair to tame frizz.

• Reduce Risk (or effect) of Alzheimer's

Alzheimer's disease is a neurological disorder in which the death of brain cells causes memory loss and cognitive decline. A neurodegenerative type of dementia, the disease starts mild and gets progressively worse. There are so many claims speculating that coconut oil can be used to cure Alzheimer. These claims have to do with ketones. Ketones are what the bodies produce when fats are converted into energy. The primary source of energy for the brain is glucose. In Alzheimer's disease, it's believed that brain cells have difficulty metabolizing glucose. But the theory is that ketones produced in our bodies when digesting coconut oil may provide an alternative fuel source to keep the brain nourished. Ketone bodies can supply energy to the brain and researchers have speculated that ketones can provide an alternative energy source for these malfunctioning cells and reduce symptoms of Alzheimer's.

• Make Homemade Soap

Soaps are usually made from 5-7 oils blended to balance cleansing/moisturizing/ and lathering properties. Coconut oil adds hardness to the soap while breaking down grease and oils effectively.

• Shaving "Cream"

Coconut oil is what I used as my shaving cream. Using the traditional shaving cream is quite frustrating because it melts away when it comes in contact with water. But with coconut oil, it bounces off the water, allowing you have a clean shave. Shave at the end of your bath or shower. The warm water opens up the hair follicles, which means you get the closest shave. Rub a small amount of coconut oil on your legs and shave using a sharp razor. For extra-soft skin, exfoliate with a body scrub before shaving. If you wish to take this further and prepare your own homemade shaving cream with coconut oil, below is the recipe.

COCONUT OIL SHAVING CREAM RECIPE

- 1/4 cup aloe vera
- 1/4 cup coconut oil
- 4-6 drops essential oil (peppermint, tea tree, lavender or a combination)

Firstly melt the coconut oil and combine it with other ingredients on the list. Stir and store in a plastic container. Apply a thin layer to skin and let sit for a couple of minutes before shaving. The aloe will soften hair while the coconut oil moisturizes your skin, helping to prevent razor burn and skin irritation. Add the essential oil of your preference. Peppermint will give a cooling sensation, lavender is soothing, and tea tree is a good antiseptic if you cut yourself.

• Deodorant

I'm very particular when it comes to my underarms. I always like them hair-free, soft, and smell free. Ever since I discovered that coconut oil works best in this department, I've ditched my usual deodorant. I like them to be soft, hair-free, and non-smelly. Coconut oil does it for me. To take this a little further I've prepared a simple recipe. Feel free to get your hands dirty!

Deodorant Recipe
- 1/3 cup coconut oil
- 2 tbs baking soda
- 1/3 cup arrow root powder
- 10 – 15 essential oils (optional)
- A small mixing bowl and spoon
- A small container for your finished product

Directions:
- Mix the coconut oil, baking soda, and arrowroot powder thoroughly in the small mixing bowl until you have an even mixture, similar to deodorant.
- Put the mixture in a small container. To use simply swipe two fingers gently into the mixture and rub on your underarms. Wait two minutes before dressing to avoid any smearing on your clothes.
- Note: Coconut oil melts when the temperatures get warmer. Some people like to keep their deodorant in the fridge during warm months.

• Lip Balm

Coconut oil works wonders as a lip balm and nourishes the lips. Honestly speaking, coconut oil has saved me huge expenses. I ditched every other lotion and went for coconut oil for a multipurpose use. You can either apply it directly on your lips or go with the recipe below.

You need:

- 1 teaspoon petroleum jelly
- 1 teaspoon coconut oil
- 4 drops vanilla extract
- 5 drops almond extract

Directions

- Put the petroleum jelly in a microwave-safe bowl
- Heat for 2 minutes, or until melted
- Mix in the coconut oil, vanilla extract, and almond extract.
- Pour into lip balm container, and freeze for 20 minutes. If there is more lip balm left over, pour it into another lip balm container.

• Dog Diet

I fed my dog regularly with coconut oil and I can see remarkable results — for their skin, digestive and immune systems, metabolic function, and even their bone and brain health. Coconut oil can also be used for itchy dogs, as it nourishes the dry, irritated, or inflamed skin that is the result of the inappropriate response to various allergens.

Below are a few uses of coconut oil for your dog.

- Coconut oil can be used to prevent and treat candida, a yeast-like parasitic fungus that can sometimes cause thrush. Its antiviral agents also helps dogs recover quickly from kennel cough.
- When you apply it topically on your dog's skin, coconut oil will promote the healing of cuts, wounds, hot spots, bites, and stings.
- Coconut oil is a powerful emollient, which helps moisturize your dog's skin. You can add it in her diet or shampoo.
- It also helps promote mobility in dogs with arthritis and other joint issues.
- Coconut oil will also help your dog reduce weight and increase their energy levels.
- Coconut oil improves overall skin health for your dog. It clears up skin

conditions, such as eczema, flea allergies, contact dermatitis, and itchy skin. My dog always gets scabby ears from excess scratching, and applying coconut oil dramatically reduced the scratching.

- Coconut oil also helps eliminate doggy breath. I normally brush my dog's teeth with coconut oil and it gives my dog awesome breath.
- Coconut oil contains antibacterial and antifungal properties, which helps to reduce doggy odour, and its pleasantly tropical aroma gives a superb scent to your dog's skin and coat.
- Do you want easy digestion and nutrient absorption for your dog? Try coconut oil. It can, however, cause them to have loose stools. To remedy that, add a few spoonful's of canned pumpkin to your dog's diet.
- Coconut oil helps prevent diabetes. It does this by regulating and balancing insulin. It also promotes normal thyroid function, and helps prevent infection and heart disease. Coconut oil is also excellent for brain health. It's a must to keep senior dogs minds from becoming cloudy.

• Coffee Creamer

To replace the usual high calorie coffee creamers, like milk and sugar, add a little coconut oil in your coffee and stir. Before you do this make sure your cup is very hot when you add it, otherwise some non-melted coconut oil might pop up.

• Antibacterial

The antiviral, antibacterial, and antifungal properties of the medium chain fatty acids/triglycerides (MCTs) found in coconut oil have been known to researchers since the 1960s. Although antibiotics are not effective in treating viruses, the lauric acid and monolaurin derived from coconut oil has been known to destroy viruses. Lauric acid is a medium chain fatty acid, which has the additional beneficial function of being formed into monolaurin in the human or animal body. Monolaurin is the antiviral, antibacterial, and antiprotozoal monoglyceride used by the human or animal to destroy lipid-coated viruses, such as HIV, herpes, cytomegalovirus, influenza, various pathogenic bacteria, including listeria monocytogenes, helicobacter pylori, and protozo, such as giardia lamblia. So next time you have a cut on your skin, apply coconut oil to prevent further infections.

• Wood Polish

Coconut oil is the best wood polish I have used. Unlike most wood polish coconut oil sinks into the wood and keeps it looking its best by giving it a pleasant shine. Start with cleaning the surface with a slightly damp cloth and dry. Follow by rubbing some coconut oil onto another clean cloth, and apply to wood in a circular motion and Let dry. To take this even further I have prepared a wood polish recipe from coconut oil.

You need

- 1/2 cup coconut oil
- 1/4 cup fresh lemon juice
- Polishing cloth

Directions

Combine the oil and lemon juice in a glass and apply with a soft polishing cloth. Polish the furniture by rubbing briskly

• Heart Disease

Much research conducted on coconut oil has proved that the oil is the secret weapon to fight heart disease. Eating coconut oil on a regular basis reduces the risk of heart attack. The medium-chain fatty acids found in coconut oil are known as saturated fats which protect you from getting heart attacks. Natural, non-hydrogenated coconut oil helps increase HDL cholesterol and improve the cholesterol profile. HDL is the good cholesterol that helps protect against heart disease.

• Lower Cholesterol

As surprising as it might seem, it's true. Coconut oil contains saturated fat and we were made to believe that a high content of saturated fat can lead to heart disease, which is linked to increased cholesterol. To add to the confusion, you'll find different types of coconut oil: virgin, refined, hydrogenated and partially hydrogenated. The former is extracted from the fresh fruit, without using elevated temperatures. Refinement often includes high heat and chemical bleaching. Processed coconut oils may not have the same health benefits as virgin. Virgin coconut oil has been repeatedly shown to be beneficial rather than detrimental on cholesterol levels and heart health. The difference is in the fat molecules. All fats and oils are composed of molecules called fatty acids. There are two methods of classifying fatty acids. The first, which you are probably familiar with, is based on saturation. You have saturated fats, monounsaturated fats, and polyunsaturated fats. Another system of classification is based on molecular size or length of the carbon chain within each fatty acid. Fatty acids consist of long chains of carbon atoms with hydrogen atoms attached. In this system you have short-chain fatty acids (SCFA), medium-chain fatty acids (MCFA), and long-chain fatty acids (LCFA). Coconut oil is composed predominately of medium-chain fatty acids (MCFA), also known as medium-chain triglycerides (MCT).

• Soothe Fly Bites

I always us coconut oil to stop the itching and swelling of insect bites or stings. I can vividly recall a certain occasion when I was bitten by cockroach. It was a horrible experience, as the area immediately got swollen and became extremely itchy. I brought out my coconut oil to soothe the affected areas and in less than 5 minutes the itching stopped and the area flattened. For severe bites apply two to three times daily, more for an even speedier recovery. Warm oil works best because it penetrates deeper.

• Acne Remedy

Coconut oil helps to promote healthy and clear skin. It is a great source of two of the most powerful antimicrobial agents found in food, capric acid and lauric acid. They are the same acids found in breast milk, which keeps newborn babies protected from infections. When these are applied on the skin, some good microbes present on the skin convert these acids into Monocaprin and Monolaurin, respectively. This helps to replace the protective acid layer on the skin. I can vividly recall when my face was filled with acne. I felt so bad about this and resorted to buying all sort of commercial creams and cleansers, which caused more harm than good, until I discovered the miraculous power of coconut oil. I immediately replaced all the oil in my house with coconut oil and started using it as my body cream. My face is now well moisturized and acne free.

• Oil/Butter Replacement

If you really want to get all the benefits of coconut oil, it's time to replace it with the other oil you use when cooking or baking. Coconut oil lends moisture, freshness, and richness to baked goods. To replace butter for coconut oil in baking, I've carefully outlined the steps for you to follow:

• Step 1
Chill the coconut oil to solidify it, especially in the summer and for recipes calling for solid butter. You may store the oil in the refrigerator to prevent it from softening or melting in the heat of the kitchen.

• Step 2
Determine the amount of butter needed by reading your recipe.

• Step 3
Measure coconut oil in a one-to-one ratio and substitute it for butter in your recipe. For example, if your recipe calls for ½ cup of butter, use ½ cup of coconut oil.

• Exfoliating Body Scrub

One of my favourite ways of using coconut oil is as a body scrub. It sure adds an extra glow and shine to your skin and it's one of the beauty secrets of most celebrities. To use coconut oil as a body scrub, it requires a little DIY technique. Below I have outlined the steps to follow.

You need:
- 1/4 cup coconut oil
- 2 tablespoons coconut milk
- 1/4 cup sugar
- 1 teaspoon lemon juice
- 1 tablespoon lemon zest

Preparation:
Melt the coconut oil in a double boiler over a low heat or in the microwave for 15 to 20 seconds. Stir in coconut milk and sugar, mixing until the sugar is thoroughly coated. Stir in lemon juice and lemon zest until all the ingredients are combined. Transfer to a glass jar. To use, massage all over dry skin before showering. Rinse thoroughly, and cleanse.

• Makeup Remover

Coconut oil also serves as a make-up remover. Well I'm not a woman, but I know this because my girlfriend uses mine to remove her makeup. I don't know who gave her that idea, but it works for her. The steps she uses are pretty basic and easy:
- **Step 1:** Scoop a small handful of coconut oil out of the jar. (Usually this will be solid, unless it is a hot day)
- **Step 2:** To turn it into a liquid, rub it gently between your palms
- **Step 3:** Smear it all over a dry face and massage it into your eyes if you've got thick eye makeup on, let it sit for a second, so everything dissolves.
- **Step 4:** To remove the makeup, grab a pad and wipe everything off.
- **Step 5:** Then rinse your face with water. There will be some coconut oil residue, so just massage it in for a moisturising treatment.

• Massage Oil

Coconut oil serves as a great massage oil and the benefits are enormous. I will list a few:
- **Healthy skin:** Coconut is rich in vitamin E, which helps nourish skin and make it smoother and softer
- **Anti-aging / anti-wrinkle:** Coconut oil is helpful in making skin look younger
- **Easy absorption:** Coconut oil is absorbed so easily that sometimes massage therapists use extra external moisturizer to make sure there is lubrication left while massaging.

- **No stains:** Coconut oil leaves no stains, unlike most oils.
- **Muscle benefits:** Massaging the body with coconut oil can help soothe and relax tight muscles. This is great if you are tired due to physical activity.
- **Anti-microbial properties:** Coconut oil has great anti-microbial properties. Medium chained triglycerides (MCTs) are considered to be great in treating various kinds of infections whether bacterial, viral or fungal.

• Nail and Cuticle Treatment

Coconut oil is perfect for nail and cuticle treatment. I got this tip from my girlfriend, while I was compiling this book. She prefers coconut oil than any other cream on the market, so I decided to add this to the list. Feel free to try it out yourself because it really works for her. I can testify to that. Rub a little into your cuticles and over/around your nails to help smooth out flaws and encourage healthy growth.

• Diaper Cream

All hail coconut oil as the perfect diaper rash cream. Search no more because you have just discovered the secret. No one likes to see their baby suffering with diaper rash. The oil has a soothing and nourishing effect, which helps heal the baby's bottom without any form of irritation and itching, making the area smooth and shiny.

Method: (Coconut Oil)
- Wash your baby's bottom properly and dry it with a towel, then apply coconut oil on the affected area with your fingertips
- Allow it to dry before putting a new diaper on your baby
- The coconut oil (an emollient oil) acts as a barrier between the skin and the faeces or urine in the diaper and prevents the rashes caused by it. This process is also used to treat the yeast diaper rash problem.

• Nipple Cream

I am not in the best position to talk about coconut as a nipple cream (as a man) but I felt I should include it. Breastfeeding can cause painful, cracked or chaffed nipples, and the best remedy for this is coconut oil. It's not a good idea to apply unknown stuff onto your nipple, because of the health of your baby. After breastfeeding gently rub a small amount of coconut oil on and around the nipple.

• Fight Inflammation

Inflammation is a localized physical condition in which part of the body becomes reddened, swollen, hot, and often painful, especially as a reaction to injury or infection. Coconut oil suppresses the effects of inflammation and helps repair tissue. It can also inhibit harmful intestinal microorganisms that cause chronic inflammation. The lauric acid in coconut oil has anti-inflammatory properties.

• Leather Polish

Coconut oil serves as a good leather polish. Clean out the dust and dirt from the leather and gently apply a small amount of coconut oil on it, rubbing it in a circular motion.

• Remove Chewing Gum

Yes, I have tried it firsthand. I don't know how…maybe because it has a way of sinking into stuff and loosening its hold. Rub it thoroughly over the chewing gum and let it sit for 2-5 minutes or longer and use a soft texture cloth or sponge to wipe the gum away. Then wash the area with a mild soap.

• Get Rid of Soap Scum

Soap scum or lime scale is a filmy layer that forms around showers, sinks, tubs, and other areas where soap and water are often present. It is caused by the minerals naturally present in water. When these minerals combine with soap, they create a sticky mixture that adheres to surrounding surfaces, slowly creating a scaly build-up that may also include body oils, dead skin, hair, and dirt. Adding oil to scum seemed counterintuitive, but I'm still amazed that it did the job perfectly. Put some oil on a rag and scrub that scum away with ease.

• Season Cast Iron Pans

The list is endless. There is a lot coconut oil can do. While writing this book I felt tempted to cut it short, but I couldn't, knowing that much would be left out if I do. Cast iron is durable and if properly taken care of, it can be passed down from generation to generation. First, make sure the pans are properly seasoned. The seasoning process helps maintain the integrity of the pan, reduces sticking, and makes clean-up a breeze. To season cast iron you will need the following:
- Cast iron pan(s)
- Coconut oil
- A dry cloth or sponge
- An oven

Do this:
- Clean and dry the pan completely.
- Preheat your oven to 325°F. Place a sheet pan or some foil over the lower rack

of your oven while the oven is cool. You can also season your pans on a grill if you prefer. This keeps the mess and potential smoke outdoors.

- Using your fingers, a cloth, or dry sponge, spread a layer of coconut oil around the inside and outside of the skillet. You can use virgin or refined. I use refined.
- Make sure the inside is coated completely.
- Place your pan face down on your top oven rack.
- Bake in the oven for 90 minutes. There is a chance of smoke, so you might want to keep your stove fan running.
- Turn off the oven, but don't open the door. Let the pan cool in the oven and then repeat as needed. Sometimes one session is all you need, but if it's a new, unseasoned pan, or one that has had the seasoning worn off, you may need to repeat the process a few times for a stronger bond.

• Bath Oil

Coconut oil also serves as a good bath oil, which gives great aroma and moisturises the skin. Below is a simple recipe to make your own coconut bath oil.

You need:
- 1 cup coconut oil
- 15 drops essential oils (I used lavender)
- Molds or ice cube trays

Do this:
- Heat the coconut oil on low heat for 1-2 minutes or until the coconut oil is completely melted, then remove from the heat and add essential oils. Mix thoroughly and pour the melted coconut oil into your molds.
- Let the coconut oil bath melts cool.
- Once cooled, pop the melts out of the molds and store them in a container in a cool place.
- If you keep your home warm (70 degrees or above) you may need to store these in the fridge or freezer so they don't melt.

• HIV – AIDS

Coconut oil does have an anti-viral effect and can reduce the viral load of HIV patients. according to University of the Philippines' Emeritus professor of pharmocology Dr. Conrato S. Dayrit. A minimum of 50 ml of coconut oil would contain 20 to 25 grams of lauric acid, which indicates that the oil is metabolized in the body to release monolaurin, which is an antibiotic and an anti-viral agent. Among the saturated fatty acids, lauric acid has the maximum anti-viral activity. Based on this research, the first clinical trial using monolaurin as monotherapy on some of the HIV patients was conducted recently. Dr. Dayrit's conclusions after the study were as follows: "This initial trial confirmed the anecdotal reports that coconut oil does have an anti-viral effect and can beneficially reduce the viral load of HIV patients. The positive anti-viral action was seen not only with the monoglyceride of lauric acid but with coconut oil itself. This indicates that coconut oil is metabolized to monoglyceride forms of C-8, C-10, C- 12 to which it must owe its anti-pathogenic activity.

• Rash Soother

Coconut oil works well with rash. It contains anti-inflammatory effects, helpful in easing the swelling and itching. Just massage a generous amount of coconut oil on the rash for about 15 minutes until the rash has cleared up.

• Reduce Dandruff

Coconut oil comes in handy when dandruff is the case. Dandruff often results due to an overgrowth of a common fungus on the scalp. To remedy this, use coconut oil 2-3 times a week to provide your hair with some anti-fungal remedy to keep the itching and flakes at bay.

• Remove Rust

Coconut oil is an excellent rust remover. To get rid of rust, simply spread a thin layer of coconut oil over the rusty area. Allow it to sit for 1-2 hours, then run warm water over the oil and wipe clean with a soft cloth.

• Prevent Split Ends

Split ends occur on the tips of a person's hair which splits as a result of dryness or ill-treatment. Coconut oil is rich in protective fatty acids that adhere to keratin easily. To remedy split ends apply a bit of coconut oil to the ends of your hair daily to reduce breakage. Keep the application to a minimal level.

• Sore throat

It's time to say goodbye to sore throat. Coconut oil is an anti-inflammatory that soothes the pain, irritation, and scratchiness of a sore throat. It is also antimicrobial, attacking bacteria, fungi, and many other viruses, so your immune system can step in and get rid of the problem faster. Swallow 1 teaspoon up to three times daily to ease the pain. To take this a little further you can make your own cough syrup with the recipe below:

You need

- 3 tablespoons fresh squeezed lemon juice
- 1/4 cup local raw honey
- 2 tablespoons coconut oil

Mix all the ingredients in a small saucepan and warm them on low heat. Remember the purpose is to melt them, not cook. Take the warm syrup with a spoon or mix it in warm water or tea and swallow. You can also melt coconut oil into tea or vegetable broth directly to reduce the soreness in your throat.

• Treat Athletes Foot

Athlete's foot is an infection also called tinea pedis, caused when various types of fungus invade the skin. It usually occurs between the toes, but it can also occur on the bottom and sides of the feet and is highly contagious. Coconut oil has powerful anti-fungal properties. These properties are due largely to the presence of lauric acid. Your body converts lauric acid into monolaurin, which has been shown to control the activity of bacteria, viruses, and fungi. To treat athlete's foot, wash the affected area and pat dry. Then apply a thin layer of coconut oil and massage properly. Make sure to wash your hands before application, to avoid further spread of the infection.

• Popcorn Topping

Yummy! When used as popcorn topping, it's simply amazing. All you need to do is melt some coconut oil and drizzle it over your popcorn, then add a little salt to it.

• Used As Toothpaste

Coconut oil serves as a perfect replacement for conventional toothpaste, which is usually full of harmful chemicals and agents. Replacing the conventional toothpaste with coconut oil is a safe alternative because it contains no foaming agent. Sodium lauryl is a foaming agent used in conventional toothpaste, which has been linked to canker sores. Coconut oil is anti-bacterial and has shown to be very effective at killing the bad bacteria in your mouth. Below is a simple recipe to make your own coconut toothpaste:

Ingredients:

- 3 tbs organic baking soda
- 3 tbs coconut oil
- 20 drops of peppermint or cinnamon oil
- 2 tsp glycerin
- A few drops of stevia or one packet of xylitol, which also fights tooth decay.

• Sunscreen

Coconut oil has been used for many years by indigenous, pacific islanders. Bruce Fife, ND, in his book Coconut Cures: Preventing and Treating Common Health Problems with Coconut Oil, explains that coconut oil, when applied to the skin protects against sunburn and cancer. Unlike sunscreen, unprocessed coconut oil doesn't completely block the UVB rays that are necessary for vitamin D synthesis. It protects the skin and underlying tissues from the damage excessive exposure can cause. Instead of burning or turning red, it produces a light tan, depending on the length of time you spend in the sun.

• Wound Care

If you have read my free e-book on putting together a natural first aid kit, I extensively wrote about coconut oil for wound care. The antibacterial and antifungal properties of coconut oil makes it ideal for minor scrapes and scratches. To take it a little further mix it with honey and apply to the area in order for healing to commence.

• Insect Repellent

Looking for an all-natural, non-toxic insect repellent that doesn't contain chemicals? I bet you are looking for is coconut oil. You can also melt the coconut oil and mix it with some essential oils like peppermint or citrus to make the perfect bug repellent.

• Bee Sting Soother

I bet you never knew that coconut oil could stop the itching and swelling of insect bites in just a few minutes? All you need do is apply coconut oil on the affected area. For an extra kick add a drop of lavender essential oil.

• Frizz Fighter

To fight frizz just apply a little amount. Pour 3 drops on your palm, rub your hands together, and smooth away a few flyways.

• Metal Polish

Coconut oil serves as a good metal polish. To polish metal, rub a little coconut oil over the metal with a soft cloth. Allow it to sit for a while, then polish.

• Moisten Chapped Nose

It's quite natural to have a chapped nose, and you don't need special medication to remedy this. But you can relive the discomfort that comes with it by applying

coconut oil. Below is a simple recipe for a chapped nose:
- 1 teaspoon coconut oil
- 3 drops tea tree oil
- Mix and apply with a Q-tip onto your chapped nose

• Coconut Oil Pulling

This is one of the best ways to remove bacteria and promote healthy teeth and gums. To do a proper coconut oil pulling use the following steps I outline below

- Oil pulling is best done in the morning, when you wake up
- Put one teaspoon of coconut oil into your mouth and chew it, so as to melt it.
- Gently swish it in your mouth and between your teeth for about 10-20 minutes, do not swallow
- Then spit out the oil and rinse your mouth with warm water.

Other Advantages of Oil Pulling are:
- Cures tooth decay
- Kills bad breath
- Heals bleeding gums
- Prevents heart disease
- Reduces inflammation
- Whitens teeth
- Soothes throat dryness
- Prevents cavities
- Heals cracked lips
- Boosts immune system
- Improves acne
- Strengthens gums and jaw

• Increase Milk Flow

A daily intake of coconut oil for nursing mothers helps increase milk supply and makes the milk more wholesome.

• Circumcision Healing

Coconut oil helps fight infections and promote healing for circumcised babies. Simply apply directly to the area.

• Eyelash Enhancement

Every lady wants their eyelashes to be long but unfortunately only a few are blessed with that. But that doesn't mean your wish can't be granted. All you need to do is apply a little coconut oil to your eyelashes every night. The protein content can encourage growth and seal in moisture, preventing brittleness and breakage.

• Preserve Eggs

To preserve your eggs, paint a thin coating of coconut oil over the eggshell. Doing this extends shelf-life and prevents degradation from exposure to oxygen.

• Grease Baking Pans

Have you ever tried taking that beautiful baked item out of the oven and watched in horror as it crumble when you try to take it out the pan? To avoid this heartbreak, grease the pan lightly with coconut oil first.

• Lubricate Kitchen Appliances

To lubricate your kitchen appliances, rub a thin layer over the blades to keep them running smoothly. Be sure to store in a cool place so the layer stays firm.

• Prevent Morning Sickness

Coconut oil can help settle a queasy stomach and keep morning sickness at bay. A tablespoon down the hatch should be all it takes.

• Cheekbone Highlighter

It will also interest you to know that coconut oil can be used to highlight your cheeks and give you that little extra glow. To do this simply apply a small amount of coconut oil on your cheeks.

• Shape Your Beard / Moustache

This one really works for man. I love keeping my beard and most of the time it look rough. Cutting it is definitely not an option. To make it appear sleek and styled, I use coconut oil. You can even go further with this and give your moustache your desired look.

• Detail Your Car

This is another amazing use of coconut oil. Apply a few drops on your dashboard or leather seats and polish. The beauty of coconut oil is that it doesn't attract dust and it smells great.

- ## Constipation Relief.

To relieve yourself of constipation try taking 1/2 tablespoon in the morning and 1/2 tablespoon after dinner. Slowly increase your intake, as if your diet does not normally feature coconut oil then you may give yourself the runs.

- ## Prevent Perineum Tears

To reduce perineum tears during childbirth apply coconut oil to the perineum. For best result apply three times a day in the months leading up to labor.

- ## Cream Foundation Base

Apply a few dollops of coconut oil on your palm mixed with your powdered mineral foundation of choice. This creates a matching cream foundation you can easily apply around your eyes and mouth.

- ## Wrinkle Buster

Wrinkles usually come with aging but you can help your skin look fresh and supple through the application of coconut oil. Do this by simply massaging coconut oil into the wrinkles and sagging skin to help bring back your youthfulness.

- ## Mascara Brush Cleaner

To get rid of mascara in your brush, simply soak it in coconut oil for 5 minutes before working with your fingers. This will make the mascara come off easily.

- ## Visibly Brighter Skin

Are you looking for brighter skin? Coconut oil can be used as an exfoliator. The combination of equal amounts of coconut oil and baking soda can make an awesome skin exfoliator. Apply this mixture to your skin in a circular motion before rinsing.

- ## Foot Exfoliator

To remove rough skin from your feet, you will need a more effective recipe. To do this mix a small amount of coconut oil with a coarser variety of sea salt.

- ## Use at Bath Time

To prevent your baby's skin from drying out, add one full teaspoon of coconut oil to your baby's bath.

• Easy to Clean Baby Bottom

Coconut oil makes your baby's bottom easy to clean. How is this achieved? Rub coconut on your baby's bottom. When it's the next time to change diapers, your baby's poop will wipe right off, with no sticking.

• Goodbye Baby Lotion

Say goodbye to baby lotion. Coconut oil is a better alternative to baby lotion. Simply mix 1/2 cup of coconut oil with raw and unrefined shea butter to form the basis of a fantastic natural alternative to baby lotion. You can also add your favourite essential oils to scent.

• Target Eczema and Psoriasis

These are both ugly diseases that leave red irritated patches on the skin and are often chronic. Coconut oil can definitely help you remedy these diseases. To do this, rub the oil on a thin layer to keep the areas moisturized and healthy, while also fighting fungus or bacteria.

• Treat Baby Thrush

Thrush is a common infection in the mouth of babies, on rashes (especially diaper rashes and rashes in moist places, such as under the chin of a dribbling baby). The antimicrobial properties of coconut oil make it a suitable treatment for thrush. Apply direct to the affected areas. This works on mamma too!

• Help Your Baby Develop

Regular intake of coconut oil can significantly increase breast milk fatty acid composition, which results in a more nourishing meal for your baby.

• Help Provide Teething Relief in Babies

If your baby is coming down with tooth pain, simply make a mixture of coconut oil and clove oil and apply it directly to your baby's inflamed gums.

• Natural Baby Massage Oil

It's time to replace your baby's massage oil witth coconut oil. If you have read to this point, I need not tell you more on the benefits of coconut oil. Coconut oil will help keep your babies skin super soft.

• Constipation Relief in Babies

There are some claims that lubricating a rectal thermometer with coconut oil and slightly inserting it into your baby's bum can relieve constipation effectively.

• Lip Exfoliator

If your lips have dry, flaky build-up of dead skin, a weekly lip exfoliation will do the trick. Below are the DIY steps to follow:
You need:
* 1 teaspoon of coconut oil
* 2 teaspoons brown sugar
* 1 tablespoon of honey (optional)

Combine all tthe ingredients and store in a jar. To use, apply a small dollop to your finger, and using circular motions apply to your lips for a minute or two.

• Maintain Lawn Mower Blades

To maintain your lawn mower blades apply a thin layer of coconut oil over your lawn mower to prevent grass clumps from sticking and jamming it.

• Hay Fever

Are you down with hay fever? Simply rub a small amount of coconut oil into each nostril for quick allergy relief. If your allergies are triggered by pollen and spores, the pollen will cling to the oil rather than enter right into the nasal passage

• Prevent Lice

Coconut oil has a way of chasing the lice away for good. To do this simply smear some coconut oil on your comb and run it through your hair.

• Aromatherapy

Mix your favourite blend of coconut oil and essential oil. Dab on your temples and the back of your neck when you feel stressed or nauseous.

• Dry Nostrils

I hate picking my nostrils when they get dried up. This can be irritating. To avoid this, I rub a little amount of coconut oil on the inside of each nostril to moisturize it. When doing this, use only a small quantity because coconut oil melts rapidly at body temperature, and too much of it can make you feel like you have a runny nose.

• Fade Age/Sun Spots

I love coconut oil for this reason. Daily application of coconut oil can help fade sun or age spots and heal skin blemishes. I wish all ladies knew this, so they would stop falling victim to the cosmetics industry..

• Bags-Be-Gone

To get rid of those dark circles that make you look exhausted, every night before going to bed rub coconut oil under your eyes.

• Soften Dry Elbows

To soften hard elbows, rub coconut oil on them morning and night to keep them supple.

• Give Your Dog a Healthy Shine

To improve your dog's skin and give their coats a lustrous shine, feed them with at least 1 tablespoon of coconut oil daily.

• Heal Wounds

To effectively heal your wounds apply coconut oil to nicks and scrapes to promote healing. Coconut oil contains anti-inflammatory fatty acids, which will help on the road to recovery.

• Soothe a Dry Canine Nose

If your dog's nose is dry or cracked rub a tad in.

• Ease Arthritis Pain

Coconut oil works well for arthritis by relieving the inflammation that is often brought by arthritis. You can do this effectively by massaging a mixture of coconut oil and aloe vera to lessen the pain associated with the swelling and inflammation that occurs in the joint. Coconut oil also adds strength to the bones and act as an agent that soothes arthritis pain in the bone and joints. Coconut oil also greases the joints in the body and help keep them loose, while leading to mobility and increased blood circulation within the joint. I recommend you massage a light coat of coconut oil on your joint after taking a hot shower.

• Flaky Scalp Treatment:

If you are suffering from itchy or dry scalp, I strongly recommend you use coconut oil. The oil helps moisturize your skin and help correct redness and irritation. Its antibacterial properties help ward off folliculitis, an infection of the hair follicles. To make your own scalp treatment, put 3 to 5 tablespoons of coconut oil in a small bowl. The amount of oil to use depends on the length of your hair. Microwave the oil for 30 seconds. Stir well, then heat for a few seconds more until the oil has melted fully. Let the oil cool a bit, then massage it into your scalp and the roots of your hair. Use a plastic comb to work the oil through your hair. Wrap your tresses in a towel or shower cap, then let the oil soak in for two hours. Finish by shampooing as usual.

• Reduce Fine Lines:

To fully understand how, you have to know that collage and elastin are the two main thing that keeps the skin firm and supple. Collagen helps make the skin firm while elastin helps the skin return to its original position when stretched. The collagen production decreases while you age and the elastin stops entirely. Hence your skin can no longer snap back to its original position. Have you ever wondered why coconut oil help heal wounds? It's because of its biologically active component known as fatty acid. Which have being shown to help increase collagen cross linking. This therefore proves why it helps reduce fine lines/wrinkles. Apply it twice daily and massage thoroughly to reduce the appearance of fine lines.

• Fight Ringworm:

Ringworm is a skin infection that falls under the category of athlete foot. It presents itself as a ring like red scaly raised bump which usually cause great itching and discomfort. To remedy this rinse the area with warm water and pat dry, after which you massage a small amount of coconut oil on the affected area. Repeat this 3 times daily for best results.

• Ease Osteoporosis:

Osteoarthritis mostly affects the trabecular bone, which is one of the two bone structures. The trabecular number refers to the measure of bone texture and structure, it marks the severity of osteoporosis. Studies conducted with rats shows that coconut oil helps increase bone volume and trabecular numbers. Also anti-oxidant activities present in coconut oil can help lessen osteoporosis caused by oxidative stress.

• Help Heal a Bruise

Coconut oil helps speed up tissue healing, repair damaged tissue and reduce time that it would take your bruise to heal and fade when used externally or internally.

• Food Poisoning Relief

Bacteria and germs have become prevalent in our society today. To remain save you should always have your bottle of coconut oil beside you. The antiviral and antimicrobial properties of coconut oil helps remedy food poisoning. When you are down with food poisoning take 2-3 tablespoon of coconut oil with a glass of orange juice.

• Tattoo Moisturizer/Healer

My very good friend just got tattooed on his left arm and for a while now he has being applying jelly oil to heal it, with no much result. I advised him to use coconut oil instead. He heeded to my advice and within a short period the tattoo was completely healed. Coconut oil helps keep your skin healthy, smooth, and moisturized and your tattoo radiant. Just apply a generous amount on the tattoo and massage.

• Dust Repellent

This seen a bit counterintuitive. Before now, you know for sure that oil is known for collecting dust, but with coconut oil it's different. Instead it gives the surface a nice lustrous polished look and keeps dust at bay. This can be applied to woods or a dashboard. To do this apply a generous amount of coconut oil on the desired surface and rub it on thoroughly, then allow to dry. Be sure to test this on small areas first to be certain that there is no discolorations.

• Cutting Board Conditioner

This works better than most cutting board conditioning oil out there. At the time of this writing, I have 2 cartoons of coconut oil which serves for multipurpose use. To condition my cutting board all I need do is wipe down the cutting board with a damp towel and then dry it. I then proceed to rubbing in some coconut oil and let it sit for about 10-15 minutes. After which I buff with a fresh cloth.

• Go-To Carrier/Base Oil

Coconut oil is mostly used as a carrier oil for lotions, lip balms, massage blends, body butter and sugar scrub. This is because of its texture and consistency, which helps hold things together.

• DIY Vapor Rub

To make a vapour rub that can be applied beneath your nose, on your chest and when you get congested. Mix peppermint essential oil with coconut oil and apply to those areas.

• On Toast

To replace butter, spread some coconut oil on for a tasty and filling snack.

• Small Motor Lubricant

I recently tried this out and it worked, so I decided to add it to the list. To lubricate small motors, mostly the ones you find in blenders, juicer and small kitchen appliances; use a small amount of melted coconut oil on it. Do not to add too much, so it doesn't solidity and have opposite effect on the motor.

• Cracked Paw Pads

I use this for my dogs, mostly when they start getting really dry cracked paw. Rub a small amount of coconut oil into the cracked paw to help them heal fast. Don't go overboard with this because you dog doesn't want its paw pads to be too silky.

• Give Plants a Shine

This is a pretty simple one, to give shine to your plant rub tiny bit of coconut oil into them to help keep the leaves looking healthy and dust-free.

• Get Rid of Cradle Cap

Cradle Cap can be caused due to overgrowth of yeast or over productive oil gland. It is a harmless condition which can result to patches of yellowish, thick, sometimes greasy scales on your baby's face. To help get rid of this, dampen your baby's hair/scalp and apply a generous amount of coconut oil to cover the affected areas. Leave it to sit for about 15 minutes to soften the scales. Then use a soft bristled baby brush to loosen and remove the patches. Then rinse off with a mild baby shampoo to remove the rest of the oil from hair.

• Improve blood circulation

Improved blood circulation can assist you if easily feel cold. Coconut oil may improve blood circulation simply by introducing it to your diet. Since LDL cholesterol can affect the viscosity of blood, and "thicken" it'. Lower levels lead to thinner blood which leads to better circulation. Start with a ½ tablespoon a day and work up to 1 tablespoon to give your circulation an energy boost.

• Ink Cleaner

I discovered this by accident. One day I mistakenly smeared my hands with ink and while trying to wipe out some spilt coconut oil on my table with the other hand, I discovered that the ink came of easily when I rubbed my both hands together.

• Breath Freshener

Are you suffering from bad breathe? Worry no more, you just found the solution. Just swish it around your mouth for 10 minute and spit out. Coconut oil helps kill the odour causing bacteria.

• Personal Lubricant

Coconut oil can be used as a natural and effective alternative to store bought lubricant. But be warned not to use it with condoms. Coconut oil is not compatible with latex, because it causes it to lose its elasticity and break down. I have experienced this first hand.

• Detangler

Coconut oil can help with those nasty hair tangle. To detangle dampen your hair well and massage oil into hair. Let it sit for 2- minutes. (Start at the bottom of the hair shaft and gently work your way up with a comb to get through the tangles.)

• Natural face mask

Instead of using mud mask to improve your complexion while not try coconut oil, which I believe is more effective than mud. To do this simply mix honey together with coconut oil. To make the mixture have a thick consistency add more honey. To take this a bit further add few drops of carrot seed oil, this helps fade scars and improve the tone of aging skin. Apply mixture to you face for 15 minutes and wash off.

• Treat enlarged prostate

Several studies have proved that coconut oil can reduce testosterone-induced benign prostrate growth in rats. Adding coconut oil to your diet may have positive effects on prostrate health.

• Urinary tract infection (UTI)

The antibacterial, antiviral and antifungal properties of coconut oil makes it very effective treatment for UTI. Simply take up to 3 table spoons of coconut oil a day until symptoms reside.

• Protozoal infections

Due to the high level of lauric acid found in coconut oil, it make it ideal in fighting protozoal infections. Simply introduce coconut oil into your daily diet to help kill off giardia (a common protozoal infection of the stomach) and other infections.

• Pre-workout supplement

I use to eat a lot of bananas for extra energy before workout. But after discovering coconut oil, I immediately made the switch. The fats in coconut oil are easily metabolized and provide a good source of energy that won't spike your blood sugar. Take a spoonful half an hour before your next workout and see if you notice a difference.

• Seizure reduction

Is your child prone to seizures? Coconut oil can increase ketone concentration in the blood which in turn can help reduce epileptic seizures

CHAPTER 10

Water Therapy and Infused Water

We all know that drinking water is one of the keys to good health, and when the case is weight loss, water can play a large role. Most of us already know about the water therapy diet, but for those who don't, I will quickly run through it before going into the main subject of this chapter, the infused water.

Water therapy diet is a fad diet promoted as a cleanse or detox. It is also known as Indian, Chinese, or Japanese Water Therapy and it's known to have a wide range of health benefits. When you embark on water therapy, at first you will experience multiple bowel movements until your body adjusts to the increased amount of fluid. The water therapy helps purify the colon and helps improve the stomach's chances of absorbing nutrients properly. It will also amaze you to know that the water therapy is one of the secrets behind glowing skin. At least that's the reason I embarked on my first water therapy. It does this by removing the toxins from the blood and improves the creation of new blood cells as well as muscle cells, and aids in weight loss. The therapy balances your lymph system, which helps you perform your daily functions, balance your body fluids, and fight infections. Drinking at least 16 ounces of chilled water can boost your metabolism by 24% in the morning, which in turn helps you lose weight.

How to do Water Theraphy

- The first thing when you wake up in the morning, before you even brush your teeth or wash your face, drink 6 cups of water at once, then wait an hour before having breakfast.

- It doesn't stop at drinking water each morning, if you want a rapid result, take it even further by drinking at least 250 – 500ml of water before each meal, and 2 hours before going to bed drink 300 - 600ml of water. All of this amounts to between 1200 – 2,450ml of water daily. I told a friend of mine about this therapy, and he decided to give it a shot. After two months he came back to recall his experience. He told me his breakfast tasted better, his skin had started to glow, and his body had become immune to common diseases like common colds and coughs.

A Japanese medical society has also found water therapy to be a 100% cure for Arthritis, Epilepsy, Bronchitis, Tuberculosis, Meningitis, Diarrhea, Throat Diseases, and many other ailments. People suffering from Arthritis and Rheumatism are advised to practise Water Therapy three times a day for one week and thereafter once a day. While following this therapy, one should drink water two hours after a meal.

Now we are done with water therapy let's take it even further and talk about the infused water. My first experience with infused water was the lemon water.

Below are a few benefits of infused water:

- I've found out that drinking infused water has greatly helped me to reduce muscle fatigue while working out, and it helps me recuperate faster after working out.

- Drinking infused water also helps to flush out toxins from your system and fills you up, so you eat less junk.

- A daily intake of infused water will help you release fat cells and keep your organs healthy while you're sweating

- It also helps improve your mood.

I believe by now you get the whole picture of what this chapter is all about and why you should drink more water. Without wasting much more of your time, let's get down to my top 6 infused water recipes.

Lemon Infused Water:

I started with lemon water, and this launched me into the world of infused waters. Lemon aids in weight loss and helps to cleanse the liver. A study published in the Journal of Clinical Biochemistry and Nutrition in 2008 found that mice given lemon polyphenols gained less weight and body fat than those not given these antioxidants. Drinking lemon water is an easy and flavourful way to replace more caloric beverages and potentially increase your weight loss. Since this is the king of infused water detox, I made an extra attempt to include its various benefits.

- The peptic fibre in lemon water is beneficial for your colon health and serves as an antibacterial agent

- Lemon is a rich source of vitamin C and other essential nutrients that help to protect the body and boost the immune system. At a point in my life, I was living an uber-unhealthy lifestyle and I almost ended up in hospital. A friend of mine told me that drinking lemon water first thing every morning can help remedy the situation. I was sceptical at first because lemon by itself is acidic. I gave it a try and it really helped to balance out my pH level.

- Lemon water helps aids digestion and encourage the production of bile

- Lemon water is a great source of potassium, calcium, phosphorous, and magnesium, which are all vital for body function

- Drinking lemon water helps dissolve uric acid and reduce pain and inflammation in joints and knees.
- Are you down with a cold? Lemon water is definitely your best bet to remedy this.
- Lemon is rich in potassium, which helps nourish brain and nerve cells
- Lemon water provides energy to the liver by strengthening the cells
- Lemon water helps remedy heartburn and balances the calcium and oxygen levels in the liver
- If beauty is your goal, then drink glass of lemon water daily. It prevents the formation of wrinkles and acne
- It maintains your eye health and helps fight eye problems
- Finally, it helps replenish the salt content in your body after a strenuous workout.

Apple Cinnamon Water Recipe:

I'm so in love with this recipe, I discovered it back in 2013 and ever since it has being my personal favourite. Please note that it's best to slice your apples very thinly, as doing so allows more juice and flavour to seep into the water. Also, for a more flavourful infusion, when drinking the water to about 2/3rds of the way down, top it with cold water and stick the jar back in the fridge for a couple of hours. The second infusion will almost be as flavourful as the first. Let's dive right into the ingredients present on our infusion. Apples are rich in antioxidant and flavonoids, which includes vitamin C and B complex. These phytonutrients and antioxidants help to reduce the risk of developing cancer, hypertension, diabetes, and heart diseases. On the other hand, cinnamon also has immense benefits, which includes lowering cholesterol, fighting diabetes, and relieving arthritis pain. It is also great for regulating blood sugar and for mental alertness. Let's jump right down to the processes involved in this.

You need:

- 1 Apple
- 1 Cinnamon Stick. (I strongly suggest you keep to cinnamon sticks, because the powdered cinnamon clogs the water)
- Water

Direction: Drop your apple slices into the bottom of the pitcher, add the cinnamon stick, and place in your fridge for about 1 hour before serving.

Lemon Lime Infuse Water

This is another recipe for rapid success in your weight loss and good health. If you read the lemon infused water section, I need not tell you about the benefit of lemon again, but I will divulge some of the benefits of lime.

- Lime is extremely good for skincare, and its natural oil is beneficial for your skin when consumed orally or taken externally. It rejuvenates your skin, while keeping its shine. Lime contains anti-oxidants, such as vitamin C and flavonoid, which helps nourish the skin.
- Lime aids in digestion. The digestive saliva floods your mouth even before you taste it. The compounds found in the fragrant oils extracted from lime, stimulate the digestive system and increase secretion of digestive juices, bile, and acids.
- Lime helps clear the excretory system by washing and cleaning your tracts. This is due to its acidity.
- Lime contains a high level of soluble fiber, which makes it an ideal diet for blood sugar regulation.
- The same soluble fibre that helps diabetics also helps keep heart disease at bay.
- Ulcers can be remedied by lemon, because of the presence of special flavonoids called limonoids, which have special antioxidant, anti-carcinogenic, antibiotic, and detoxifying properties that stimulate the healing of peptic ulcer.
- When uric acid builds up in your body, it can sometimes lead to arthritis. Lime helps the body get rid of arthritis.
- Taking a glass of infused lime water can greatly help you lose weight. The citric acid present in lime is an excellent fat burner.
- Lime contains high potassium content, which helps rid the body of toxic substanced that gets deposited in the kidneys and the urinary bladder.
- Piles are uncomfortable conditions that occur in the anal region and can result in bleeding and great discomfort. Lemon water helps to eradicate the root cause of pile.
- Gout are mostly caused by excess free radical and toxins accumulation in the body. Regular intake of lime water helps detox the body from these harmful substances.
- If someone is suffering from fever, limes and lime juice can be of great importance.
- Now we are done with the benefits of lime let's dive straight into making our sinful lemon and lime infused water. Firstly, be sure you have only organic produce.

You need:
- 1/2 Lime
- 1/2 Lemon
- Water

Direction:
Cut the lemon and lime thinly. I advise that you cut the rinds off because it might cause a slight bitterness in the infused water. Put the slices of lemon and lime into the pitcher, add water and ice, and place in your fridge.

Lemon Cucumber Water:

Cucumber water is loaded with plenty of vitamin and nutrients, which is an anti-inflammatory food, while lemon helps boost immunity. They are both packed antioxidants like vitamin C, which increase collagen and elastin production that results in younger skin. Cucumber also has anti-inflammatory properties that prevent water retention and silica to promote healthy connective tissues. It also contains an anti-inflammatory flavonol called fisetin that appears to play an important role in brain health and helps maintain a healthy weight. Washing your face with cucumber and lemon water helps refresh the skin, closes pores, and helps prevent oiliness. It will also interest you to know that placing a cucumber slice on the roof of your mouth may help to rid your mouth of odor-causing bacteria.

You need
- 1/2 lemon, thinly sliced
- 1/4 cucumber, thinly sliced (about 4 inches)
- 2 cups of ice
- Water

Direction:
 Slice your lemon and cucumber and add them in a large pitcher followed by ice and water. Put it in your fridge and let it sit for a few minutes. Pour in a glass and enjoy. Once your water is down to only ¼ full refill with water. It will still retain its flavour as before.

CHAPTER 11

Marvellous Miracles of Epson Salt

I had Epsom salt in my kitchen for close to a year with knowing the immense benefits it holds. The sad part was that there was a period when I suffered from severe muscle pain, so I visited the hospital to seek medical solutions, and ended up with drugs prescriptions, which cost me a fortune. A month later I discovered that having an Epson salt bath was a better alternative, and I had it all along in my kitchen.

Epsom salt is made up of naturally occurring minerals, magnesium and sulphate. These minerals help in numerous ways, like flushing toxins from the body, sedating the nervous system, reducing swelling, and relaxing the muscles.

Magnesium regulates the activity of more than 300 enzymes in the body, and the lack of it may lead to blood pressure, hyperactivity, heart problems, and other health issues.

Below are the marvellous miracles of Epson salt.

• Take a nice relaxing bath after a hard day's work.

Boy, there's nothing relaxing like taking a relaxing bath with Epsom salt after a hectic day. Perhaps this is one of the best uses of Epson salt. The magnesium relieves minor aches and pains. Studies also show that magnesium and sulphate are easily absorbed through the skin. Sulphates play an important role in the formation of brain tissue, joint proteins, and the proteins that line the walls of the digestive tract. To do this, simply pour a cup of Epson salt into your warm bath, let it dissolve, then immense yourself deep inside. This is the perfect home spa treatment.

Below are the health benefits:

- Having an Epson bath helps improve heart and circulatory health, reduces blot clots, reduces irregular heartbeat, and lowers blood pressure.
- Having an Epson bath helps flush toxins from your cells, and also helps to ease body pain while eliminating harmful substances from the body.
- It also helps reduce inflammation to relieve muscle cramps and pain.
- Since Epson salt is rich in magnesium, it helps maintain proper calcium levels in the blood.
- Since magnesium is a natural stress reliever, it helps bind adequate amounts of serotonin, which is well known for its role in the brain where it plays a major part in mood, anxiety, and happiness.
- It also helps improve oxygen use and absorption of nutrients.
- It also helps improve formation of joint proteins, mucin proteins, and brain tissues
- Whenever I'm hit with a migraine headache, an Epson bath is a must go-to remedy as it has a way of soothing the headache.

Foot soak / pedicure

Epson salt makes for an invigorating foot soak. I use it to remove odours and soften my feet. To do this simply add ½ cups of Epson salt to a large bucket of water and soak your feet for as long as you want. Then rinse and pat dry.

Soak sprains and bruises

It will amaze you that Epson salt can also be used to soothe swelling and bruises. Simply start by adding 2 cups of Epson salt into warm bath and soak yourself.

End constipation

I read in a book that one of the best natural supplements one can take to relieve constipation is magnesium. Since Epson salt is rich in magnesium it makes sense for it to do the job fine. I know what's going on in your mind now! Have I tried it? Yes I have, and it works. Simply start by dissolving a teaspoon in a glass of water and drink up – this should soften your stools.

Hangover cure

Epson salt is a lifesaver and always good to have in the house. I can remember vividly on a certain occasion when I over-indulged in alcohol, I was so messed up that I needed to snap out of it as soon as possible because I had another important engagement. A glass of diluted Epson salt saved the day. This was made possible because Epson salt contains sulphates, which help break down toxins and flush them out faster. But do note that this remedy calls for drinking a lot of water.

Face cleaner

Epson salt also serves as a good face cleanser. To use it in this department simply mix half a teaspoon of Epson salt with your regular cleansing cream and massage onto the skin. Rinse with cold water and pat dry.

Skin exfoliator

You can also use Epson salt to exfoliate your skin. Start by massaging a handful of Epson salt over your wet skin. I suggest you start with your feet all the way to your face, after which have your bath and pat dry.

Remove excess oil from hair

This is one thing baking soda and Epson salt have in common – the ability to soak the excess oil from your hair. To do this, simply add 9 tablespoons of Epson salt to ½ cup of your hair shampoo. Proceed to applying just 1 tablespoon of to your hair, let it sit for a while, then rinse. You can take this further by pouring lemon juice onto your hair, leave for about 10 minutes, and then rinse off.

Remove hairspray

To remove hairspray, create a mixture of 1 cup Epson salt, 1 cup of lemon juice, and one bowl of water. Leave the mixture for about 24 hours then pour the mixture into dry hair and let it sit for about 20 minutes. Rinse and pat dry.

Hair volumizer:

To add extra volume to your hair, combine equal parts of deep conditioner and Epson salt together. Heat this mixture until it's warm enough, then apply the warm mixture to your hair and leave on your hair for about 20 minutes before rinsing off.

Eye wash

It will amaze you that Epson salt also helps with eyes too. To ward off eye defects such as cataracts, conjunctivitis, or sties, dissolve a small portion of Epson salt in water and use it as an eyewash. Alternatively, you can apply it on a white towel and use it as a warm compress

Relieve minor irritation

To remedy mosquito bites, bee stings, mild sunburn, poison ivy, and other minor irritations start by making a cold compress by soaking a washcloth in cold water that has been mixed with Epson salt, and gently apply to the affected areas.

Relieve gout

The magnesium content of Epson salt helps combats inflammation, which helps decrease swelling as well as reliving pain. Simply pour some Epson salt into your hot bath and soak the affected joints.

Remove blackheads

Blackheads appear on the skin, usually the face, and it's when the pores of the skin become blocked. Blackheads can be very annoying and irritating to live with. When squeezed they spread rapidly and mostly can't be left lying around. They don't just look good. Thank goodness I discovered a way to get rid of this pesky skin condition. Start by mixing a teaspoon of Epson salt with three drops of liquid iodine and half a cup of boiling water. Leave this concoction to cool down, then dab it onto the blackheads with a cotton wool bud. Repeat this severally until the blackheads come away. Follow this up with astringent.

Make grass greener

As a young boy I was curious to see my mum spread a gallon of diluted Epson salt on our lawn, even though I didn't know the purpose of her doing so, but I didn't hesitate to ask why. She smiled at me while patting my hair and said, "You see how green our lawn is… have you ever wondered why?" At that moment it dawned on me that the salt water was responsible for the amazing job. This is because Epson salt adds the needed magnesium and iron to your soil. To try this for yourself simply add 2 teaspoons to one gallon and spread it over your lawn with a garden sprayer.

Insecticide spray

Epson salt can also be used in lawns and gardens to get rid of plant pests naturally. Simply spray the salt water all over your garden.

Beautiful roses

If you grow roses this tip is for you. For faster growth, add a tablespoon of Epson salt every week to the soil around the rose bushes before watering.

Bigger, better, and more produce

Using Epson salt on your farm can lead to bigger, better, and more produce. I can still vividly recall how granny mixed 1 teaspoon of Epson salt in a gallon of water. Using a garden sprayer, she then sprayed it over her peppers, tomatoes, and blooms, which usually results in bigger yields.

Get rid of raccoons

Annoying bandits! Are you tired of seeing these annoying guys that eat just about anything and loiter around everywhere? Simply take a few tablespoons of Epson salt and spread it around your cans. This should keep these pesky guys in check as they don't like the smell.

Clean bathroom tiles

Cleaning your bathroom tiles with the usually ordinary soap and detergent won't give you that sparkling look. To eliminate those stubborn stains that won't come off, mix an equal part of Epson salt with your liquid soap, then dab it onto the stubborn stain and scru. Trust me, this will do the job just fine.

Remove burnt foot from pot and pans

There is no chore as tedious as trying to remove burnt food from pots and pans. Sometimes it just won't come off and you have to live with it. But with Epsom salt it comes off effortlessly. Simply scrub your pan with ¼ tablespoon of Epsom salt and warm water. This does the job pretty well.

Regenerate your car battery

This is one of the reasons I love to leave Epson salt in my vehicle trunk. You can give your car battery a little more life by dissolving an ounce of Epson salt in warm water to create a paste. Add the paste to each battery cell and watch the magic happen.

Help kids sleep better

To help your kids sleep better, start by adding a cup to your kid's bath before bed. This will help your child sleep peacefully.

Get rid of slugs

Do you have slugs in your garden or on your patio? Sprinkle Epson salt to deter them.

Sore muscles and splinters

To treat sore muscles and splinters, start by making a cold compress by soaking a cotton washcloth in cold water that has been mixed with Epson salt. Apply a compress to the affected areas. Alternatively, create a paste of Epson salt by adding a teaspoon to a cup of hot water and stir until it dissolves, then chill the solution by putting it in the fridge for about 20 minutes. Clean the skin and apply the paste on the affected area.

CHAPTER 12

Home Remedies for Constipation

Let's face it at some point in our lives, each and every one of us has suffered from constipation. It is a very common digestive disorder that affects people of all ages, which leads to difficulties in passing stools.

I can still recall one certain period in my life. I suffered from chronic constipation. I had difficulties pooping for close to five days. I felt so ashamed to share this with anyone because it's not something you talk about with people. I got some drugs from the pharmacy, which didn't work. Lastly, my girlfriend recommended I try some natural alternatives. Constipation can lead to bloated abdomen, acidity, loss of appetite, bad breath, headache, depression, acne and mouth ulcer. Some of the major causes are poor diet, insufficient water intake, and irregular defecation habits, weakness of abdominal muscles, haemorrhoids, stress, laxative abuse and intake of certain medication. Below, I have collected some home remedies to help with constipation; I hope you find them interesting.

Take castor oil.

Castor functions as a stimulant laxative, which lubricate the bowels without absorbing any moisture from the walls of your intestine. Which allows the stool slip away with less stress. Try as much as possible not to take too much of castor oil, because it can cause unpleasant side effects like abdominal cramps, dizziness, fainting, nausea, diarrhea, skin rash, shortness of breath, chest pain and tightness in the throat.

You need this:
- Castor Oil
- A glass of juice

Directions:

When buying castor oil, check it the following is written on it: cold pressed/processed, virgin, 100% pure, and USP food grade. This is to ensure that you are getting a high-quality product. Determine the proper dosage by reading the instruction written on the label or by the recommendation of your doctor. Take the castor oil on an empty stomach for maximum result. Alternatively, since castor oil is known for its bitter and unappealing taste, you can dilute it with the juice of cranberry, orange, prune or ginger. After which you will experience a bowel movement. Castor oil should not be taken at night because the laxative effect is usually very rapid.

Baking soda

I love baking soda. It's a vital ingredient for most home remedies. Baking soda has numerous benefits, which I wrote in the previous chapters. It contains bicarbonate which makes it very potent for constipation. Bicarbonate encourages air to come out of you one way or another while relieving pain from pressure. It also balances the pH level of your stomach while helping things pass through your gut.

Get this...
- One teaspoon baking soda
- 1/4 cup warm water

Directions

Mix ¼ cup of water with one teaspoon of baking soda. And gently gulp down the mixture.

Lemon

Lemon juice helps stimulate the digestive system, while allowing your stool to pass away easily. This remedy is one of the simplest home remedies for constipation.

Get this
- Lemon
- Glass of water

Directions
Drink the natural lemon juice mix with a little warm water. Alternatively, you can add a pinch of salt and honey to the mix. Lemon juice should be drank first thing in the morning on an empty stomach. Keep to this remedy for a few days to see the result.

Aloe Vera

Aloe vera plant is known for centuries for its health, beauty, medicinal and skin care properties. The name was derived from the Arabic word "Alloeh" meaning "shining bitter substance," while "vera" in Latin means "true." 2000 years ago, the Greek scientists regarded Aloe vera as the universal panacea. The Egyptians called Aloe "the plant of immortality." Today, the Aloe vera plant has been used for various purposes in dermatology. Aloe vera contains 75 potentially active constituents: vitamins, enzymes, minerals, sugars, lignin, saponins, salicylic acids and amino acids

Get this-
- Two tablespoons of pure aloe gel or one cup of aloe vera juice

Directions
Mix two tablespoons of pure gel with fruit juice and drink in the morning, OR drink one cup of aloe vera juice as needed.

Fennel Tea

Powdered fennel seed act as a laxative. It stimulating effect helps maintain muscle contractions that occur in your digestive tract, thereby promoting proper excretion through the stimulation of gastric juices and bile production. The roughages also help clear your bowels.

Get this
- Fennel Seed
- Mortar and Pestle
- Boiling water

Directions
Pound one cup of fennel seed using mortar and pestle, this help release the volatile oils and compounds. Pour freshly boiled water into the bruised seed, allow it to steep for 10 minutes. Sieve out the liquid content and drink. Doing this will relieve your constipation in few hours.

Figs

Constipation can cause you to have hard or big stools that are difficult to pass. Which can make your bowel movements painful. Constipation can result from factors such as a low-fiber diet. Figs are rich in fiber content and acts as a natural laxative.

Get this
- Almond
- Dried Figs

Directions
- Soak two to three almond and dried figs in water. Peel off the almond and grind them ingredients. Take the paste with one tablespoon of honey at night.

Honey

Honey acts as a mild laxative, and it is very beneficial in relieving constipation

Get this
- Honey
- Lemon juice
- Warm water

Directions
- Mix one tablespoon of honey and lemon juice in a glass of warm water and drink the mixture on an empty stomach first thing in the morning. Alternatively, Consume just two teaspoons of honey three times daily

Flaxseed

Flaxseed is rich in fiber and omega-3 fatty acids, with a high laxative property, which is useful for constipation.

Get this
- Flax seed
- Glass of water

Directions
Add one table spoon of flax seed in a glass of water and allow it to steep for about two hours. Then drink the liquid content daily before bedtime. Alternatively, you can eat two to three tablespoons of ground flaxseed with a glass of water. Your constipation should be over by morning.

Grapes

Grapes are very effective in relieving constipation. They contain insoluble fiber which helps produce regular bowel movements

Get this
- Small bowl of grapes
- ½ glass Milk

Directions
Drink a glass of fresh grape juice or eat a few grapes. Alternatively you can put a few seedless grapes in milk. Boil it for a few minutes and drink the solution. Use the particular remedy for mostly children suffering from constipation

Fiber

I recommend eating high fiber rich food because fiber is a natural laxative, which increases the water content of your stool. It will also help your bowel movement more quickly and smoothly through the colon. Expert recommends that you get at least 20 to 35 grams of dietary fiber each day.

Some choices for increasing your fiber intake include:
- Berries and fruits with an edible skin, such as apples and grapes.
- Dark, leafy green vegetables like collard, mustard, and beet greens, Swiss chard. broccoli, spinach, carrots, cauliflower, Brussel sprouts, artichokes and green beans.

- Beans and other legumes such as kidney, navy, garbanzo, pinto, lima, and white beans, lentils and black-eyed peas. Whole, unprocessed grains, such as brown rice, popcorn, steel-cut oats, and barley. Seeds and nuts such as pumpkin, sesame, sunflower, or flax seeds, almonds, walnuts and pecans

Prunes

Prune juice is rich in a substance known as dihydrophenylisatin, a laxative that aids muscle contractions. Secondly, it contains a number of different sugars like sucrose, fructose and sorbitol that help in drawing fluid into the intestines, thus helping the passage of waste out of the body. Studies has shown that prune juice greatly helps in increasing the volume of fluid that remains in the waste passing through the intestine while also causing contractions that aid bowel movement. The fiber in prunes also stimulates the muscles of the intestines and peristalsis. This motion helps for absorption and processing of nutrients. Which in turns get your intestines back into working order by absorbing water to helps break through the blockage and cures constipation

Get this
- Prune
- Juicing Machine

Directions
Juice the prunes with a juicing machine, and take the juice. 100 grams of prune juice has 6.1 grams of sorbitol. This remedy should start working within few hours.

Molasses

Molasses contains several essential vitamins and minerals like magnesium, iron, copper, calcium, potassium, manganese, selenium which all helps prevent constipation. The mineral content that helps remedy constipation in molasses is magnesium. It also has natural laxative property that aids in alleviating constipation, by ensuring regular bowel movement. Molasses helps remove toxic waste from the body. Its alkaline property helps balance the stomach pH, which in turns helps for proper stool formation an regulate bowl movements

Get this
- Blackstrap molasses
- A cup of milk (optional)
- Prune Juice (optional)
- Peanut Butter (optional)

Directions

Eat one teaspoon of blackstrap molasses before bed time. You can as well mix it with milk, fruit juice or prune juice. Alternatively, mix two to three tablespoons of molasses with an equal amount of peanut butter and eat in the morning.

Avoid cheese and dairy products.

Lactose is found in high quantity in products like cheese and dairy product, which many people are allergic to. This can further cause gas, bloating and constipation for some people. Sometimes cutting out cheese, milk, and other dairy product can be the simple remedy for constipation. But except yogurt, because yogurt contains probiotics such as Bifidobacterium longum or Bifidobacterium animalis has been proven to promote more frequent and less painful stool passing.

CHAPTER 13

Home Remedies for Menstrual Cramp

According to Mayo Clinic, Menstrual cramps (dysmenorrhea) are throbbing or cramping pains in the lower abdomen. In which the body sheds the lining of the uterus (womb), and is then passed through a small opening in the cervix and out through the vaginal canal.

Many women experience menstrual cramps just before and during their menstrual periods. The pain experienced with menstrual cramp differs with different women. For some, it's just a slight discomfort but for others, it can be severe enough to disrupt a full day's function. Some of the pain usually experienced are aching pain in the abdomen, pain in the hips, lower back, and inner thighs, feeling of pressure in the abdomen.

According to webmd.com, menstrual cramps are caused by contractions of the uterus, in which the uterus, the hollow, pear-shaped organ where a baby grows, contracts throughout a woman's menstrual cycle. If the uterus contracts too strongly, it can press against nearby blood vessels, cutting off the supply of oxygen to the muscle tissue of the uterus. Pain results when part of a muscle briefly loses its supply of oxygen.

Below are home remedies that can help you cure menstrual cramp.

Ginger:

My mom always advised my sisters to use raw ginger each they experience a menstrual cramp. This remedy stuck to my head till adulthood. On a particular when my girlfriend was experiencing severe menstrual cramps, it came right out of my mouth, she gave it a try, and her menstrual cramps eased. Ginger plays helps lower the level of the pain causing prostaglandins and helps the fatigue associated with premenstrual syndrome.

Directions:
You can choose to eat it in its raw state or cooked. Alternatively boil few slices of ginger, add honey and a pinch of salt. Leave to simmer for 4 minutes. Drink twice daily. If the ginger you have is in dried powder or grated form, add ½ teaspoon into a cup of boiling water and leave for 3 -5 minutes. Drink this three times daily for best results.

Cinnamon:

Cinnamon is another potent remedy to soothe menstrual cramps. The anti-inflammatory, antispasmodic and anticoding nature helps relieve menstrual pain.

Directions:
You need to start by making a cinnamon tea by adding a ¼ tablespoon of cinnamon powder into a glass of water. Leave it for about 5 minutes to dissolve completely in water. You can add honey to sweeten the portion, then gradually sip it slowly. Keep in mind that it's best to drink this portion one to two days before your period starts, in other to prevent cramps in advance

Chamomile Tea:

A study published in the Journal of Agricultural and Food Chemistry has found that chamomile tea contains compounds that may help fight infections due to cold and relieve menstrual cramps. Drinking chamomile tea can significantly increase the level of glycine. Higher levels of glycine have being shown to relax the uterus, which explains why the tea relieves a menstrual cramp.

Directions:

Pour one tablespoon of dried chamomile powder in a cup of boiling water. Stir properly and allow to steep for 5 – 10 minutes. Strain the tea. At this point you can add lemon juice or honey, the choice is up to you. Then gently sip. I highly recommend you drink at least two cups of chamomile tea a day during the week before your period.

Parsley:

Parsley also does a great job. But just that it's not my usual recommendation. Parsley is rich in apiol. A compound which has been shown to stimulate the menstrual process and relieves your cramps.

Directions:

Start by washing your parsley thoroughly, after which you add it into the container of your choice. Then pour in one cup of boiling water. Let it steep for about five minutes. Strain the mixture and drink the tea immediately.

Peppermint:

Peppermint is a widely used remedy for menstrual cramps owing its ability to the fact that it's a natural muscle relaxer and appetite suppressant.

Directions:

You can either use peppermint leaves or its powder. Add any one of your choice into a cup of boiling water. Don't allow it to heat; moderate heat is needed. Remove from heat and let it steep for about 3 – 5 minutes. You can also add honey, it all depends on your choice. Drink this tea 1 -2 times a day for instant relief. Alternatively drink two cups of peppermint or wintergreen tea a day. Also suck on mint candy on and off during the day.

Basil:

Basil has a natural painkiller called caffeic acid which relieve the pain of menstrual cramping.

Directions:
Start by putting two tablespoons of basil leaves in a cup of boiling water. Allow it to steep for about 5 minutes and cover it tightly until it comes to room temperature. Then drink ½ – 1 cup hourly to get rid of the pain.

Heat or Hot Compress:

This heat compress is usually the first remedy I recommend to my clients when they are in dire need for a quick fix. Warm compress relieves menstrual pain as the pain is a result of clogged blood. When you do warm compress, you are melting the clogged blood resulting in a smooth flow. To do this use hot water bottles or hot water bags on your abdominal area and lower back where it hurts the most. Doing this will reduce the intensity of the cramps by relieving the muscle tension.

Exercise:

Exercise is another great way to lessen menstrual cramps, and also get to rip other numerous benefits it offers. Exercise releases endorphins which act as a natural pain killer and mood lifter. Frequent exercise helps relieve menstrual cramps. If you don't have the time to hit the gym, I suggest you practice some yoga moves at home or with some friends. Yoga helps increase the blood flow to your reproductive organs, relieves stress and gives you the needed relaxation. Try the restorative yoga poses which are best for reliving menstrual cramp

Prevention Tips

- Instead of looking for quick fixes for menstrual cramps, it pays to avoid it beforehand. Below are a few things to bear in mind.

- To prevent painful bloating during menstruation, you need to drink as much water as possible. Drinking warm or hot water will increase blood flow to your skin and relax cramped muscles

- Eat foods rich in water content. Foods like cucumber, watermelon, berries, pineapple, and celery to increase hydration and give you needed relief.

- Eat water-based foods or fruits such as celery, watermelon, cucumber, berries, and lettuce to increase hydration and get relief from cramps.

- Foods rich in calcium should also be eaten to reduce muscle cramping during menstruation. Foods like milk, sesame seed, almond and green leafy vegetables.

- Eat foods rich in vitamin B6 such as brown rice to reduce bloating.

- Consume at least two tablespoons of flaxseed. During this helps reduce pros taglandin production (responsible for menstrual pain or cramps) in the body due to its herbal properties. Consume two tablespoons of flaxseeds daily for best results.

- Reduce the intake of coffee. Decaffeinated coffee intake, more especially.

- Cut down on the consumption of alcohol

- Cut down on salt intake before your period begins

- For added omega 3 fatty acids, eat cold-water fish or take fish oil supplements. This helps inhibit the production of prostaglandins.

- The use of intra-uterine devices (IUDs) as a method of birth control should be avoided. These devices can increase menstrual cramps.

- Swallow 2 teaspoons of apple cider vinegar (ACV) after each meal

CHAPTER 14

Basic Beauty Routine

Like every other thing in life, you need to understand the fundamentals, before you can get it right. Beauty is not an exception. Before we dive right into the subject of skin care and beauty, we need to understand rudiments first. I had the opportunity to sit one on one with Isabella. Isabella owns one of the biggest beauty clinics in Lagos, which she has run for close to 5 years. Her skin is flawless and always glowing. She is one of the most beautiful women I have seen. Below is her basic beauty routine.

❝ A basic skin care regimen comprises of cleansing, toning, and moisturizing. Firstly you have to remove the dirt and bacteria. Then you refine your tissue and then keep your skin hydrated" says Isabella.

Cleansing:

She recommends you start by cleaning your face at least twice daily. If you have a mild skin, go for a mild non-alcoholic cleanser. But it you have a harsh skin go for a little tougher product to get a good result. Isabella resonates with nature, and her personal favorite beauty ingredient is the lemon. She confessed to me that lemon is the secret behind her light and bright skin. She even made me buy a cartoon of lemon. These days I use it on a daily basis to remove my age long black spots and boy it works. For what it's worth my face needs to look pretty good before I can sell you beauty remedies.

Other natural cleansing alternatives she uses are listed below:

- **Tomato:** Tomato also makes for a good cleanser. Cut tomato into two halves and rub one part over your face and neck. Let it sit for 15 minutes and wash off afterward.

- **Lime:** Lime can also pass for a great cleanser, and it can be used as a facial scrub.   Simply extract the juice, with the aid of a cotton swab cleanse your face with it. Do not overuse lemon as a scrub. You can do it once every three days.

- **Buttermilk:** Buttermilk also does a great job. To use is as a cleanser simply take diluted buttermilk and dab on your face. Leave it for fifteen minutes and gently wipe off with a cotton swab.

- **Honey:** I just love honey. Unfortunately, is can be hard to get the original one. But I always have my way of getting 100% honey. To cleanse your face with honey; start by wetting your face with warm water. Pour a reasonable quantity on your palms and rub it together. Using those honey palms of yours rub it on your face while massaging it on your face in a circular motion. Leave it for 10 minutes for a deep cleansing effect. Then wash off with warm water and pat dry.

- **Aloe Vera:** Aloe vera when used as a face cleanser has a cooling effect and calms your skin. You can use Aloe Vera on its own or jazz it up with other ingredients. Isabella gave me a wonderful cleansing recipe you can use with aloe vera.

you will need
- ¼ cup of Aloe Vera,
- Two Tablespoons of almond oil
- Two tablespoons of rose water,
- 5 – 10 drops of lavender oil
- One capsule of Vitamin E oil.

- **Directions**

Mix up all the ingredient. Apply the mixture on face and massage in a circular motion. Leave in on your face for about 15 minutes. Rinse off with warm water and pat dry.

Yogurt, Oatmeal, and Cucumber:

Isabella said that this remedy is intended for those with dry skin. It very useful in removing impurities from your skin while hydrating it. For this cleanser, you need two tablespoons of cooked oatmeal, ¼ of cucumber and two tablespoons of plain yogurt. After you are done combining all three ingredients in a bowl. Apply on your face and massage it in a circular motion. Let it sit for 15 minutes before rinsing it off.

Un-Boiled Milk:

Dip a small cotton swab into a one tablespoon of unboiled milk and apply on your face, while massaging it in a circular motion. Leave on your face for 15 minutes before rinsing off with warm water.

Avocado:

Isabella said that this cleanser is most suitable for those with sensitive skin or those with dry skin. It has a soothing effect that can be used to reduce redness and irritations on your skin. Simply mash up avocado in a small bowl and apply to your face. Leave it for 10 minutes and wash off with warm water. Pat dry.

Tomato, Milk, and Lemon Juice:

This cleansing recipe will help balance the skin and help remove dead skin cells and impurities, and can be used for any skin type, but don't overuse it.

Get your ingredient together,
- One ripe tomato,
- Two tablespoons of milk and
- Two tablespoons of lemon juice.

Direction

Mix them all together using a food processor, till you get a smooth consistency. Start by washing your face with warm water. Apply the paste on your face and neck, while you massage it in a circular motion. Let it sit for 15 minutes. Rinse off with warm water and pat skin dry.

Toning:

After cleansing, you need to tone up your skin to remove all the trace of dirt, makeup or cleansers that might be left out after cleansing your face. Isabella's best natural toner is the apple cider vinegar, which she believes is the best. Make sure that when applying the toner, you touch areas like crevices around the chin and crevices around the nose.

Moisturizing:

Isabella says it necessary to moisturize your skin if you have dry skin. Moisturizing your skin forms a thin coating or film over your face that protects you from the direct effect of sunlight. Moisturizing helps keeps your skin smooth and supple throughout the day. Isabella's is one woman that will never use a store bought moisturizer. It's funny how most people believes she is using the most expensive moisturizer in the market. But she gave me her cute little secret, which is virgin coconut oil. Coconut oil is full of collagen supporting lauric acid, which is easily absorbed by the skin, and can be used on oily and acne prone skin. I have written extensively on coconut oil in the previous chapter. To use coconut oil as a moisturizer, place few drops on your fingers, press the fingers of your both hands on the middles of your forehead and gently work it slowly outwards, making sure it covers around your jawline and chin. Make sure to avoid contact with your eye and massage thoroughly so as to get absorbed by your skin.

Additional Facial Skin Care Tips:

Below are some other skin care tips from Isabella.

Drink plenty of water to keep your skin hydrated:
She advises that you drink plenty of water in a day at least eight glasses of water and eat fruits and vegetables rich in water content. Foods like cucumber and pineapple. She told me that drinking at least four cups of water upon waking up in the morning keeps your skin glowing. I smiled when she said it because it's something I do every day for glowing skin.

• Protect your face from harmful UV rays:

Early morning sun is good for you and anything apart from that damages your skin, so try as much as possible to protect yourself face from direct sunlight. She advises that you moisturize your face with coconut oil. It goes a long way in protecting your skin from the direct effect of sunlight.

• Exfoliating Facial Scrub:

Facial scrubs can help your skin become brighter and softer while buffing away dry, dead cells on your face; while revealing the fresh cells underneath. But this should be done in moderation. It stimulates the skin which results in improved blood circulation. If you are facing blemishes and dark spots problem, it is ideal exfoliate your face regularly, says Isabella. Doing this removes the dirt on your face which reduces the skin imperfections and contributes towards a flawless skin. Follow the habit of using facial scrub two to three times weekly.

• Avoid touching your face:

Isabelle advises that you try your best to avoid touching your face. When you touch your face always, it increases the tendency of scanning for irregularities, which might also lead to picking at blemishes and running a high risk of worsening them. It can even cause acnes scarring. Also, our hands come in contact with millions of germs, via doorknobs, shoelaces, and smartphones,w and when we touch our face regularly, this germs makes it to our face and can lead to unwanted breakouts.

• Remove your facial hair:

She advises that you keep your eyebrow line neat, and remove hairs from the upper lip and chin. You can use a tweezer to pull out unwanted hair. If you feel the tweezer is time-consuming, use an epilator. A device which pulls out multiple hairs on the face at once. You can also try waxing

• Lips care:

Most women believe that the best way to care for the lips is to wear lipstick. Your lips should be kept moisturized. She told me that sugar goes a long way in caring for the lips. It helps remove dead cells and rejuvenate your lips. Run sugar-water solution on them, and use a moisturizer on them.

Keep a stick of lips moisturizer handy and use it whenever you need to. However, do not use too much of chap-stick, as your lips can get addicted to the chemicals that heal / prevent chapped lips, and they will stop producing natural oil. Which will make you entirely dependent on the chap-sticks.

• Nourishing Face Mask:

Isabella recommends you use a homemade facial mask at least once a week to keep your face glowing.

CHAPTER 15

Home Remedies For Snoring

More than anything, I hate snoring. I once had a partner who snores. I tried all I could to make her stop, but nothing seems to be working. The usual night elbow I give her on the ribs didn't seem to stop her. Leaving the room for the sitting room didn't do much good either.

I thought about quitting the relationship because I definitely can't face the reality that I would spend my whole life in this torture. It was either she stops snoring, or am done. All I wanted was a sound sleep at night. We talked about this issue and how to put an end to it. Together we started seeking out various remedies for snoring. Below are what we gathered. We applied a few of them and got the result we needed. Even though the relationship ended in the long run, but I thought I should share this with you guys. It can be of help to those who needs it.

Lifestyle Remedies for Snoring

Various unhealthy lifestyle habits can cause snoring. When does habits are stopped, snoring can significantly reduce.

• Lose weight:

Losing weight can dramatically help you stop snoring. More fat around your neck region squeezes the internal diameter of your throat. Which is more likely to collapse when you sleep. I will advise you go on a regular juice fast, to lose the extra pounds.

• Avoid alcohol and sedatives:

Avoid Alcohol and sedatives. They relax the tissue in your throat, causing it to expand and block off the airway, which results to snoring.

• Clean your bedroom often:

A dirty and dusty room may give you serious allergies, which can lead to snoring. Allergens like pollen, dust, animal dander, and other unseen irritants can cause congestion and irritate your airways, so it mandatory you clean up the room properly.

• Stay hydrated:

Secretions in your nose and soft palate become stickier when you are dehydrated, which causes more snoring. Try and have at least eleven cups of water in a day.

• Don't smoke:

Smoking can significantly irritate the mucous membranes which lead to throat inflammation. This narrows down your airway and causes nasal congestion.

• Exercise regularly:

Two times in a week is moderate. Exercise can help you in maintaining a consistent sleep schedule as well as assisting with weight loss. When we get regular exercise, your body get toned, including the muscle in our throat.

To tackle snoring, it's best to diagnose the cause first. Some people do snore with their mouth closed while others snore with their mouth open. Learning to distinguish the kind of snoring will help you remedy the situation:

• **Closed-Mouth Snoring:** This indicates that your tongue is the major cause of your snoring and that exercise is needed to help eliminate snoring

- **Open-Mouth Snoring:** This is usually caused by sinus trouble or bad posture and can be corrected by addressing those issues

- **Snoring from any position:** indicates apena or requires medical treatment

Use a Tennis Ball

This remedy that worked well for my ex-girlfriend. For some people, breathing becomes disturbed when they sleep on their back. Sleeping on your back allows gravity to shift your tongue tissues of the soft palate into your airway. Which in turns obstruct the airflow from your nose or mouth to your lungs. It's best to maintain a sideways position while sleeping to prevent snoring. One way to do this is to make use of the tennis ball. By attaching a tennis ball to your back, it makes it impossible to sleep on your back due to its discomfort.

Materials needed
- One tennis ball
- Pocket of an old shirt
- Needle and thread
- Scissors

Directions
Carefully cut out the pocket of an old unused shirt. Sew the pocket into the mid back region of your pyjamas top (make sure it's well tight so that the ball wouldn't fall off). Drop the tennis ball into the pocket before bed. (The tennis ball will cause a slight discomfort, whenever your partner wants to roll over)

Use a Backpack

Another way to avoid not sleeping on your back is to place a backpack filled with bulky items like a solid baseball or softball over your shoulders.

Materials needed
- Backpack
- Any Bulky Item

Directions
- Fill the backpack with bulky materials like softball or baseball.
- Place the backpack over your shoulder. This way, if you move your back, the discomfort from the ball will cause you to shift over to your sides

Elevate Your Head

Sleeping on an elevated position can help take some pressure off your airways, improve your airflow and place your tongue and jaw into a better position

Materials
- Several Pillows
- Books

Directions
- Sleep on multiple pillows or by putting your books under your pillow

Gargle with Peppermint

If allergies cause your snoring, peppermint is an option for you. Peppermint is anti-inflammatory which helps reduce the swelling of the membranes in the lining of the throat and nostrils. Doing this promotes easy and smooth breathing. Peppermint remedy works well for temporary snoring.

Materials needed
- 3-4 drops of peppermint oil
- A glass of water

Directions
- Add two drops of peppermint oil to a glass of water. Gargle the mixture before going to bed.
- Do not swallow the mixture
- Repeat till you get the desired result

Inhaling steam

Nasal congestion is one of the main reasons behind snoring. One of the best ways to reduce nasal congestion is by inhaling steam.

Materials
- Hot boiling water in bowl
- Eucalyptus Essential Oil
- Towel

Directions
- Pour hot water into a large bowl and add 3-4 drops of eucalyptus essential oil.

Hold a towel over your head and inhale the steam deeply through your nose for about 10 minutes. Repeat this process daily, till congestion clears

Nettle Leaf Tea Remedy for Snoring

When allergies are your primary cause of snoring, nettle tea is one of your best remedies. Sometimes, when sinus passage get inflamed due to allergies of the upper tract infections such as cold or sinusitis, your snoring might increase. Nettle tea is well known to reduce congestion by inhibiting the release of histamines. Histamines are the inflammatory substance that is triggered by allergens. Due to the bioflavonoid content of nettle tea, it opens up the sinuses and stabilizes white blood cells that make histamine.

Materials
- One tsp- Dried nettle leaf
- One cup - Boiling water

Directions
- Add one tablespoon of dried nettle leaves to one cup of boiling water. Leave the mixture to steep for five minutes, then strain it. Drink the warm tea just before bedtime. Drinking two to three cup daily during the allergy season can help prevent snoring

Garlic Remedies for snoring

If your snoring is due to sinus, garlic is the remedy for you. Garlic helps reduce mucus build-up in the nasal passage as well as respiratory inflammations. Some herbalist says that garlic can treat snoring due to sleep apnea because it helps soothe and reduce enlarged tonsils as well as inflammation in the respiratory system.

Directions
- Chew on a few garlic cloves and drink water before bedtime. The odor might also disturb your partner. Alternatively, you can crush garlic and mix it with butter to make as toast.

Mint Tea

Mint contains menthol which reduces mucous from your lungs and also reduces inflammation of air passage.

Materials
- 8-10 mint leaves
- Hot water
- 1-2 teaspoon of Honey

Directions
Put the mint leave in a cup and pour in the hot water. Let it steep for 5 - 10 minutes and strain the mixture. Add honey to the mix and take the cup near to your nostrils and inhale the minty steam coming out of the hot cup of tea. Gradually sip the mint tea

Turmeric
Turmeric is a potent antibiotic and antiseptic agent that helps treat inflammation and reduce heavy snoring. Turmeric is best used with milk to treat snoring.

Materials
- Turmeric Powder
- A glass of milk

Directions
- Add two teaspoons of turmeric powder to a glass of warm milk and drink the mixture 30 minutes before bed time. Repeat daily, till you get needed result.

CHAPTER 16

Amazing uses of lemon for beauty

Just as I was about to send my manuscript to my editor, I receive a last minute email from my buddy. The email was on the beauty uses of lemon. Thank God this email came, because I would have hated myself if this book was published without this remedy.

I can't believe I left it out, this is something I do almost all the time. Lemon is not only good for your overall health, it also plays a huge role in the beauty department. If have read this book closely, you will see several remedies that calls for lemon. Below are a few beauty uses of lemon.

- ## Blackhead:

The simplest way to get rid of black head if you don't have the time to prepare any strenuous home remedy is to slice a lemon, using the second half, scrub it thoroughly on your face. Lemon have anti-bacterial properties that will help get rid of your black head in no time. Just repeat this before going to bed every night till blackhead vanishes.

- ## Elbow and knee bleacher:

This remedy reminds me of my sister. She had dark knees and spent most of her time scrubbing lemon on her knees. Funny enough this solution worked for her. If such is your case, feel free to try it out.

- ## Canker sore treatment:

Lemon can be used to heal canker sore quickly. I thought that baking soda is best alternative, but lemon offers equal healing effect. Pour a few drops of lemon on canker sore to help them heal faster.

- ## Clarifying moisturizer:

Lemon on its own can help clear and brighten up your skin, but when combined with coconut water makes for an effective clarifying moisturizer. Make a mixture of coconut water and lemon, moisturize your face with it. The coconut water will help hydrate your skin and lemon will help clear and brighten your complexion.

- ## Cleansing wipes:

One of the best DIY cleansers you can make is lemon mixed with tea tree essential oil in 6 ounce of water. Use a cotton swab and soak in the solution, then wipe your face with it.

- ## Get rid of wrinkles:

Fine lines and wrinkles can be a big issue for many. This remedy is not a quick fix for it, but with continuous application it will surly do a great job in getting rid of wrinkles and fine lines. To do this, Mix two drops of lemon juice with a drop of almond oil and a tablespoon of honey till it forms a thick consistency. Apply the solution on your face and let it sit for about 15 minutes. Afterwards rinse off with cool water and pat face dry. Be careful not to get this solution into your eyes, because it wouldn't be funny if you do.

• Teeth whitener:

Looking for a teeth whitener that works? Try baking soda and lemon juice. Make a paste of baking soda and lemon juice and apply it to your teeth with a clean A-tip. After then use your toothbrush to scrub your teeth and rinse off. This a cheaper alternative than wasting some cool cash in the dentist office

• Lighten / brighten Your Skin:

Don't expect quick result with this, but consistence is the key. Lemon contains citric acid that have natural lightening properties. The vitamin C content in lemon is also a great antioxidant for neutralizing free radical and boosting collagen production. Which implies that it can help lighten age spot and dark spot. The way I use it is to cut lemon into two half's, the other half I used it to scrub my face. I let it sit for about 15 minutes before rinsing it off.

• Lips exfoliator:

Lemon can be used as a lips exfoliator. I tried this a couple of time, and I can bet it's better than most store bought lips exfoliator. Simply pour a few drops of lemon juice on your lips before bedtime and leave it overnight. Wash off early in the morning upon waking up.

• Hair Lightener:

As surprising as it seems, lemon helps lightening hair. You can do this by applying before you expose your hair to direct sunlight. It can also be used to treat dry scalp and dandruff.

• Tone up your Skin:

To tone up your skin with lemon juice, mix two tablespoons of lemon juice, one tablespoon of witch hazel, one tablespoon of water and 2 tablespoons of vodka. This solution is very efficient for oily skin to get rid of excess oil. Remember to rinse and pat dry afterwards.

• Nail strengthener:

Lemon can save you the few bucks you waste in manicures. It can be used to remedy dry, brittle and yellow nails. The best way to use it in this fashion is to mix lemon juice with olive oil, then soak your nails in side for about 15 minutes.

- ## Shine Eliminator:

Lemon is perfect for reducing excess oil.

- ## Moisturize Your Skin:

  - To moisturize your skin mix equal parts of lemon, olive oil, and honey. Apply to the dry areas of your skin. Leave it for 15 minutes and then rinse off with water. It moisturizes even the driest of skin.

- ## When using lemon I want you to take note of these few pointers.

  - Avoid exposure to direct sun light with lemon juice on skin

  - If you notice any irritation or dryness, dilute the lemon with water immediately.

  - It is always best to moisturize your skin after using lemon juice. Because it is acidic and can dry out skin it not moisturized

  - Be careful not to apply lemon onto open, cuts and bruised wounds. The acid content in lemon stings and if it touches your wound, you wouldn't find it funny

CHAPTER 17

Home Remedies for Dandruff

Few years ago I worked with a hair care company that specializes in the production of anti-dandruff products. The hair care company own a hair clinic where they attend to various hair defects, most notably dandruff and hair fall. What seemed striking to me was how much women were willing to pay to get rid of dandruff. Most of the products used in the clinic contained labelling like tea tree, coconut oil, and aloe vera.

On several occasions, I visited the factory where these products were manufactured; I never got to see any of those essential oils mentioned on the labels; just a bunch of machines mixing chemicals.

So I figured out they used false labeling to lure people into believing that their products were made from nature's ingredients.

That's the whole truth about these commercial industries. They are motivated by the amount of money they make not by the individual needs. It saddens me that most people fall prey to their antiques.

Dandruff can be caused by several factors ranging from dry skin, irritated oily skin, not shampooing often enough, yeast, sensitivity to hair care products and other skin conditions. Below are some of the best home remedies for dandruff.

Lemon for Dandruff

Lemon juice works well to get rid of dandruff. It contains anti-fungal properties that help prevent dandruff-causing fungus. Lemon has a healing property which soothes the irritated scalp, reduces itching, clears the scalp of dead cells and discourages the growth of fungal. Due to its acidic nature, it balances the scalp's pH level and prevents dandruff. The juice of fresh lemon contains essential antioxidants and vitamin which is helpful in promoting healthy scalp and hair.

How To Use Lemon For Dandruff.
- Squeeze the juice of one fresh lemon directly on scalp, with the help of a lemon wedge. Leave it to sit for about 20 to 30 minutes. Then wash your hair off with clean water and shampoo.

- If applying lemon directly on hair is too concentrated for you. Then start by diluting the lemon juice with 1 tablespoon of rose water. Apply the mixture on your scalp and massage thoroughly. Then, leave it on your hair overnight.

- Lemon can be combined with coconut oil to make an excellent dandruff remedy. Start by mixing two tablespoons of warm coconut oil with one tablespoon of lemon juice. Apply the mixture on scalp and massage thoroughly. Leave it on your hair for about an hour and wash off with a mild shampoo. Lemon and coconut oil have an anti-bacterial property which helps to fight dandruff causing fungus and promotes a healthy scalp.

Baking Soda for Dandruff

Baking soda does a lot of things. Getting rid of dandruff is one of them. When regularly used on the scalp, it can help clear dandruff. For what it's worth, baking soda help removes excess oil, dirt and dead cells from the scalp. Most people use it as a dry shampoo, to help suck oil and dirt from hair and scalp, leaving hair soft and shiny. Due to its alkaline nature, it helps balance the scalp's pH. Baking soda comes in an excellent texture, which can act as a scalp exfoliator, to get rid of dead cells and grime present on the scalp.

How To Use Baking Soda For Dandruff.

- *Mix baking soda with rosewater to make a paste.* Apply the paste on scalp and massage for about 5 minutes. Massaging baking soda on the scalp helps to create a scrubbing effect which loses all flaky dandruff and dead cells. Wash off with a mild shampoo afterwards

- *Baking soda can be mix with lemon to form an excellent combination.* Mix juice of freshly squeezed lemon with baking soda to form a paste. Apply the paste on your scalp and let it sit for about 5 minutes. Wash mild shampoo and rinse off. Do this twice a week to rid your hair of dandruff naturally.

- *Another great combo is the baking soda and vinegar.* Mix baking soda with apple cider vinegar to form a paste. Apply the paste on scalp and massage thoroughly on the scalp. Wash off with a mild shampoo. Do this twice a week for best results.

Aloe Vera for Dandruff

Aloe Vera is another remedy widely used for dandruff and also in Ayurvedic medicine and other beauty products. When applied to your scalp, it penetrates deep into the hair to kill bacterias and clean your scalp. Aloe Vera is anti-fungal, which makes it very potent in killing dandruff causing fungus while minimizing flaking of the scalp. Its antiseptic properties soothe the scalp and reduce itching. It is a natural moisturizer, prevents drying up of scalp and locks in moisture.

How to use Aloe Vera for Dandruff

- *Cut open the aloe vera and scrape out the gel.* Apply the gel directly on your scalp and spread it. Massage on hair for about 10 minutes and let it sit on your hair for about 30 minutes. Wash off after that with a mild shampoo and water. Do this thrice a week to completely get rid of dandruff and promote healthy hair.

- *Aloe vera gel and lemon is also a great combination.* Start by mixing equal part of aloe vera and fresh lemon juice in a clean bowl. Massage the mixture into the scalp, with the aid of your finger. Leave it to sit for about 30 minutes before washing off. Do this twice weekly for maximum results.

- *Aloe vera and baking soda can also be combined to make a thick paste for dandruff.* Apply the paste on the scalp, using a brush distribute on hair. Let it sit for 30 minutes before rinsing off. Baking soda scrubs the scalp while removing dead cells and preventing the growth of fungal.

Ginger for dandruff

Ginger is also used to get rid of dandruff. When the juice of ginger is applied to the scalp, it removes dandruff from the root of the hair and encourages healthy hair growth. Ginger is anti-fungal which helps kill fungus and cleanses the scalp. It's essential vitamin and mineral helps promote strong, shiny and healthy hair. Ginger contains active volatile oils that enhance blood circulation, cleans scalps and leaves a fresh fragrance on the hair.

How to use ginger for dandruff

- *Mix two tablespoons of ginger juice, three tablespoons of sesame oil and a dash of fresh lemon juice.* Apply the mixture on your scalp and massage thoroughly. Leave it on your scalp for about 15 to 20 minutes. Wash and rinse off with a mild shampoo. Use this thrice a week for maximum result.

- *Ginger and Aloe Vera can also make a great portion for dandruff.* Start by mixing two tablespoons of aloe vera gel with one tablespoon of ginger juice. Apply the mixture on your scalp and massage thoroughly for a few minutes. Leave the mixture for 20 minutes before rinsing off.

- *Ginger and lemon juice also make a potent mix for dandruff.* Mix equal parts of lemon juice and ginger juice in a small bowl. Apply the juice on your scalp and massage thoroughly. Leave it on your scalp for about 15 to 25 minutes, before washing off.

- *Coconut oil can also be mixed with ginger juice to remedy dandruff.* To do this, combine fresh ginger juice with one tablespoon of warm coconut oil and one tablespoon of olive oil. Apply the mixture on your scalp and massage thoroughly. Leave it for 30 minutes on hair before washing off. This warm oil therapy should be adhered to at least twice weekly to get rid of dandruff.

Apple Cider Vinegar and Dandruff

Apple cider vinegar is another well-known natural remedy to get rid of dandruff. It contains mallic and acetic acids with other powerful enzymes which kill fungus and bacteria in the hair. When applied to the scalp will help maintain a healthy pH balance. The acidity also helps in reducing itchiness and flaking, while giving shine and volume to your hair. When applied to hair it also helps open and cleanse clogged pores

How to Treat Dandruff with Apple Cider Vinegar

- Apple cider vinegar can be used with Fenugreek to form a potent paste for dandruff. Grind fenugreek seed to make a paste, then add few drop of ACV and mix thoroughly to make a consistent paste. Apply the paste on your scalp and leave it for 20 minutes. Wash your hair with mild shampoo.

- You can also use a diluted form of apple cider vinegar to spray on your hair. To do this mix equal part of ACV and water. Pour the mixture into a spray bottle and spritz on your hair and scalp. Be very careful to avoid your eyes and ear. Cover your hair with a shower cap and leave it for 20 minutes before washing off.

- ACV can also be mixed with tea tree oil, olive oil, and lemon juice to make a remedy for dandruff. To do this add ½ cup of ACV, five drops of tea tree oil, ½ teaspoon olive oil and juice of half lemon into one cup of distilled water and mix. Pour the mixture into a spray bottle and shake thoroughly. Spray on scalp and cover hair with a shower cap. Leave it on hair for 30 minutes before you wash off with a mild shampoo.

CHAPTER 8

Alternative Treatment for Canker Sore

Canker sore is an irritating and annoying ulcer that occurs on the surface of the lips. If you have experienced it, you know what am saying. Also known as aphthous ulcer, they are the small and shallow lesion that develop on the soft tissues in your mouth or the base of your gum. They are very painful and can make eating difficult, but they aren't contagious. While most of them tend to vanish after two weeks.

Causes
- Viral infection
- Stress

- Hormonal fluctuations
- Food allergies
- Menstrual cycle
- Vitamin or mineral deficiencies (especially iron, folic acid, or vitamin B-12)
- Immune system problems
- Mouth injury

Baking Soda

- Due to its alkaline property, it helps neutralize the acidity of the sore and soothe the pain and inflammation, while fighting off the bacteria in your mouth.

Get this:
- Baking soda- 1 tsp
- Warm Water- 1 Glass

Directions:
- Make a paste of baking soda by adding a little warm water to a reasonable amount of baking soda.
- Wash your fingers and use it to apply the paste on the affected areas.
- Let it sit for a few minutes, then rinse with lukewarm water.
- Repeat this three to four times a day
- Alternatively, you can mix two teaspoons of baking soda in warm water and rinse your mouth with it. Repeat this for four to five times daily

Onion

Onion is rich in sulfur, which helps heal cancer sore and soothe the pain and inflammation.

Get this:
- Onion

Directions:
- Make a paste of onion and apply it directly to the sore area.
- Let it sit for about 10 minutes (Make sure the juice get absorbed into the sore)
- Repeat this for two to three times daily
- Alternatively, you can eat raw onion daily to remedy cancer sore

Coriander

Coriander does an excellent job in treating canker sore. A friend of mine used it and recorded remarkable results. I strongly do recommend you try it if you have canker sore. Due to its anti-inflammatory, antiseptic and anti-fungal properties its quiet effective in reducing pain and discomfort associated with canker sore.

Get this:
- 2 tbsp Coriander leaves
- 1 glass of Water

Directions
- All you need to do is add the coriander leaves into water.
- Boil the leave in the water for a couple of minutes
- Strain the liquid out and let it cool for some minutes
- Rinse your mouth with the liquid
- Repeat this three times a day for best results

Hydrogen Peroxide

Yes, this works. Hydrogen peroxide is antiseptic and can helps kill the bacteria in the canker sore. There by activating the healing process.

Get this
- Cotton ball
- Hydrogen Peroxide

Directions:
- Soak the cotton ball with a generous amount of hydrogen peroxide
- Gently apply this to the sore until it "fizzes."
- Repeat this three times daily, for best results

Sea Salt & Honey Rub

Putting salt on canker sore can be a painful experience, but it helps to remedy canker sore. Salt owes it's healing ability to the fact that it helps draw the fluid from a canker sore and also speed up the healing process. Honey is antibacterial and adding honey, makes it easy to apply salt.

Get this
- 1/2 teaspoon of sea salt
- Organic raw honey

Directions
- Make a paste of salt and honey, by adding a little quantity of honey to salt, just enough to stick together.
- With clean fingers, apply the paste directly to the sore and allow it to sit for 5-10 min utes
- Repeat this 2 – 3 times a day for best results

Aloe Vera

Aloe Vere is another remedy you should try out. My mom told me about this one, and I saw it work for a friend. Aloe Vera owes its healing ability from its inflammatory and antibacterial properties. It helps ease the pain and inflammation associated with canker sore and speeds up healing process.

Get this
- Aloe Vera

Directions
- Scrap out the gel from aloe vera and place it directly on the canker sore. Or you can as well rinse your mouth with aloe vera juice. Three teaspoons of aloe vera gel can be taken daily.

Coconut Oil

I love this oil. When this book is out. I plan on starting an e-commerce business, selling essential oils. Mostly coconut oil. Coconut oil is anti-inflammatory and antimicrobial which helps remedy canker sore.

Get this
- Coconut Oil
- Cotton Wool

Directions
- Soak your cotton wool with coconut oil. Use the cotton wool to press onto the canker sore. Leave it to sit for about 5 minutes. Repeat this three times daily for best results

Cayenne Pepper

Another great alternative is the cayenne pepper cream. I discovered about this on a web forum, and further research proves that it works. Cayenne contains capsaicin that temporarily numbs the nerves, thereby giving you instant relief from the pain and inflammation.

Get this
- Cayenne Pepper

Directions
- Make a paste of cayenne pepper by mashing the pepper and mixing it up with a little water.
- Apply the paste directly on the affected area. You will feel some irritation at first, just endure, the remedy is working. Repeat this three times a day for best results.

Sage Tea Rinse

Sage is another great alternative for canker sore. Its calming properties give instant relief to the pain and inflammation associated with canker sore

Get this
- Sage leaves
- One cup of water

Directions.
- Add some sage leaves into boiling water and leave it for 10 minutes.
- Allow the mixture to cool off.
- Then sieve out the mixture and rinse your mouth with it.
- Alternatively, you can apply the powdered sage leaves directly on the canker sore. Repeat this three times daily for best results.

Honey

You can always rely on honey to do the job. Honey is antiseptic, soothing and has antibacterial properties. Canker sore pain can be severe at times and honey is the best fit for this.

Get this
- One teaspoon of honey
- Turmeric Powder

Directions
- Collect some of the honey with your finger and gently dab it on the canker sore. It will hurt at first, but endure. Leave it to sit for about 10 minutes. Alternatively, make a paste of honey by mixing it with turmeric powder. Apply the paste directly on the sore. Leave it to sit for a few minutes. Then rinse your mouth with salt water. Repeat this process three times daily.

Tea Tree

Tea Tree is also very useful in the treatment of canker sore because of its antiseptic and antibacterial properties.

Get this
- Tea Tree

Directions
- All you need to do is add eight drops of tea tree oil into a glass of water.
- Rinse your mouth thoroughly with the solution.
- Repeat this several times a day.
- Alternatively dilute two drops of tea tree in a one-half tablespoon of water and apply the mixture directly on the canker sore. Do this three times daily

Chamomile Tea Bag

Chamomile Tea is very effective in the treatment of canker sore. It contains a chemical compound called bisabolol which has antiseptic properties and has been proven to help reduce inflammation and speed up the healing process.

Get this
- One bag of chamomile tea
- One cup of water

Directions
- You need to soak the chamomile teabag in warm water for about 3 minutes.
- Remove from water and place directly on the sore for about 5 -10 minutes.
- Do this twice daily for best results.

Dehydrate your canker sore with Milk of Magnesia.

Milk of Magnesia is a white suspension of hydrated magnesium carbonate in water, used as an antacid or laxative. It is applied in the treatment of constipation. It comes in tablets and liquid form.

Get this
- 1 tsp Milk of Magnesia
- Cotton swab

Directions
- Soak the cotton swab into one teaspoon of milk of magnesia.
- Dab it on the canker sore and let it sit for 5 – 10 minutes.
- The magnesium hydroxide will dehydrate the canker sore and help speed up the healing process. Repeat this 2-3 times daily.

CHAPTER 19

Get Rid of Dark Circles Naturally

Few months ago, while in India. I gazed at the mirror and was furious on the amount of dark circles on my beneath my eyes. Before then, I stayed awake most nights writing my book and drinking caffeine. (Guessed that was the cause of my sudden old man look).

I had to do something to get rid of them. I look like I have the whole problems in the world. The worst was that I have a photo-shoot coming up the next few weeks. So I can't be caught dead looking like a zombie. The interesting thing about India is that sourcing for ingredients to use for your remedies is easy. In India peeps hardly use over the counter beauty products – spices of different kinds are littered in every nook and cranny. If you are still wondering what dark circles are, they are dark blemishes seen around the eyes. They are as a result of blood vessel beneath the eyes becoming visible. Having dark circle gives you a tired look, even when you are not tired. Other factors that can lead to a dark circles are hereditary, allergies, anemia, sickness and poor diet. Dark circles is common among older people. If you are young and have dark circles, then it's time to do something about it. Don't worry, read on, you will know what to do. I have listed all the natural remedies for dark circles I learnt from India.

Cucumber:

If you are serious about clearing your dark circles, you should consider using cucumber. A friend of mine once told me about this, but I took it with a pinch of salt, not until another friend confirmed his claims. I recommended it to a client, after a while she came back with positive Feedback. Cucumber has skin lightening effect and is an excellent astringent and skin toner.

To use cucumber, cut the cucumber into slices. Place the slices in the refrigerator for 30 minutes. Then remove and place them on the affected area for about 10 minutes. Wash off the area and pat dry. Repeat this process twice daily for a week. Alternatively, you can mix equal amount of cucumber juice and lemon juice. With the aid of a cotton ball apply the solution on the affected area and leave it for about 20 minutes. Wash off and pat dry. Do this every day for a week; you will be amazed on how your dark circle will begin to vanish. If you don't have lemon available, you can make do with just cucumber juice. Dip two cotton swab into cucumber juice and place it on top of your eyes. Let it sit for about 15 minutes, then wash off with plain water. Do this daily. Trust me you will see positive results.

Rose Water:

When the idea of this post came to my mind, I knew the best person to call was Jessica. Jessica is a natural beauty expert, most of the things I write about beauty; I learnt from her. So I asked Jessica what natural remedies she recommends for removing dark circles. Her answer was the Rosewater. She recommends you dip two cotton balls into rose water and place them on your eyelids. Let it sit for about 10 minutes. Repeat this twice daily for at least two weeks for best results.

Almond Oil:

Am thrilled to add almond oil on this list because I have seen it work, not just on anybody, but on me. I used almond oil under my own eyes for close to one month, before going to bed. Over time, the skin under my eye became lighter. To try this yourself, place a few drops of almond oil on your fingers and massage it around your eyes. Do this every night before going to bed and wash it off while taking your morning bath. Do this consistently and gradually, the dark skin will fade away.

Tomato:

Jessica's second remedy for dark eyes is tomato juice. Although I knew that tomato is used for various beauty remedies. It never occurred to me that you can also use it for dark circles. To make it more potent, mix one tablespoon of tomato juice with on tablespoon of lemon juice. Apply the mixture on the affected area. Let it sit for about 10 minutes. After that, rinse off with cold water. I suggest you do this twice daily for best results. An alternative way is to create a concoction of tomato juice, mint leaves, and lemon juice – with a pinch of salt. Take this concoction orally, twice daily for about a week

Raw Potato:

I have always known about potato's ability to remove dark circles because I have always seen my mom use it. When Jessica mentioned it, I wasn't surprised. The idea is to apply potato juice on the affected area. It will be much easier if you have a juicing machine. Juice the potato to extract its liquid. Dip two cotton balls in the juice and place it on the dark circles. Make sure that the juice covers the affected area. Let it sit for about 15 minutes, then rinse off with cold water. Try this out twice daily for best results. You can take this recipe a bit further and add cucumber juice. Repeat all the steps outline above.

Turmeric:

My first encounter with turmeric root was during my stay in India. Ever since then, turmeric never seizes to amaze me. Turmeric always appears in most Indian Ayurveda practice. I have taken the time to study this herb. Its anti-inflammatory and antioxidant properties help clear dark circles. Add few drops of pineapple juice to two teaspoons of turmeric powder. Apply this paste on the dark circles and let it sit for at least 10 minutes. Then wipe off with a damp cloth.

Lemon Juice:

Lemon is an excellent source of vitamin C. It will interest you to know that lemon had skin lightening properties. Curious to know how? Cleanse your face with lemon juice for a long period. Your face will gradually become lighter and brighter. To remove dark circles, with the aid of a cotton swab apply lemon juice under your eyes. Let it sit for about half an hour, wipe it off with a damp cloth. Repeat this process twice daily for best results. A second alternative is to mix one tablespoon of lemon and two tablespoons of tomato puree to form a thick paste. Add a pinch of gram flour and turmeric powder. Apply the paste around your eyes. Let it sit for 15 minutes before rinsing off with clean water. Repeat this process at least thrice weekly.

Mint Leaves:

Mint leaves are one of the most effective remedies to consider when removing dark circles. You got to love mint leaves because it gives a cooling effect to the eyes, while soothing and refreshing your eyes. To start, crush five mint leaves and apply them around your eyes. Let it sit for about 10 minutes. Then wipe off with a cold cloth. Dear one, just be careful, so it doesn't touch any sensitive part of your eye. An alternative way to use mint leave is to add it to your tomato puree to form a thick paste. Apply this paste on the dark circle. Let it sit for 10 minutes. Rinse off with cold water and pat dry.

Apple:

Apple also does a great job in getting rid of dark circles. It is an excellent source of tannic acid. And plays a huge role in skin lightening and also rich in vitamin B, C, and potassium. Apple helps nourish skin around the eyes. To use this remedy, cut your apple into slices and place them under the eyes. Leave for 20 minutes and wash off with cold water. You can also mash the apple and apply under eye for the same effect.

Chamomile Tea Bags:

You can also try out chamomile tea bags. There are various speculations it works too. Although I have never tried it out myself, but reliable sources confirmed its potency. Soak chamomile tea bags in hot water and rinse it with cool water. Place them on your eyes and let it sit for 20 minutes. Wash off the areas with plain water. Alternatively, tea bags can also be to achieve the same effect. This is due to the caffeine and antioxidant present in tea; which helps get rid of dark circles and puffiness under eyes by shrinking the blood vessels and reducing fluid retention. The tannins also helps decrease swelling and discoloration. Chill two used green or black tea bags in the refrigerator for 2 minutes. Place them over your eyes and leave for about 15 minutes. Remove the tea bag afterwards and wash off. Do this once or twice daily for a few weeks.

Hey buddy, now you know all the remedies to use, I have a few pointers I need you to know. Knowing all these remedies and still not changing your unhealthy lifestyle wouldn't do you much good. You wouldn't want the dark circle to keep coming back! Would you?

- Water intake plays a huge role to avoid the occurrence of dark circle. Drinking at least 15 cups of water daily will help prevent dehydration that can also lead to dark circles.

- Always consume your vegetables. For me, I get more vegetable into my body through juicing. The soluble fiber helps clear toxins in the body

- Don't be like me – have enough sleep, at least 7 to 9 hours per day. Lack of sleep is the major cause of dark circles.

- People with a sweet tooth are more prone to have dark circles. Avoid eating too many sweets.

- Does your work give you stress? If you answered yes to this question, please resign, it's not worth it. Find the work you love. well, that's just my opinion.

- Smoking and doing junk can also lead to dark circles. Try as much as you can to avoid those.

- Avoid the use of too much makeup or chemical bleaching around your eyes.

- Reduce your salt intake. When salt accumulates in your body. It leads to excessive fluid retention, which in turns leads to under eye puffiness.

- Try as much as possible to get enough vitamin E into your daily diet – feel free to supplement. Vitamin E helps cure dark circles.

- Increase your intake in food rich in vitamin C. these foods will keep you fresh and make your skin glow every day. Foods like oranges, lemon, and grapefruit.

CHAPTER 20

Homemade honey facial masks

Avocado Honey Mask for Dry Skin

The two key ingredients in this mask are used in several beauty remedies. Honey helps retain moisture and the oil in avocado treats dry patches.

Ingredients:
- One tablespoon avocado, mashed
- One teaspoon honey
- ½ teaspoon heavy cream

Directions:
Mix honey, avocado, and heavy cream thoroughly till it forms a thick consistency. Apply the mask on your face and massage in a circular motion. Leave it for about 15 minutes before rinsing off with warm water.

Tightening Egg White Mask

This is my personal favourite, maybe because the ingredients involved are readily available. Raw honey helps kill bacteria on the skin. Lemon juice is acidic and helps reduce age spot; while egg white is perfect for oily skin and can be used for tightening and firming up of your skin, while warding off fine lines and wrinkles

Ingredients
- One egg white
- One teaspoon lemon juice
- One teaspoon raw honey

Directions
Mix all the ingredients together and apply it on your face. Gently massage on your face. Leave it to dry up for about 20 minutes before washing with warm water.

Anti-Aging Flaxseed + Honey Mask

Flaxseeds are high in antioxidants and are anti-inflammatory. They are rich in Omega 3 fatty acids which are quite good for your skin. When combined with honey, serves as the perfect exfoliate, which is ideal for fighting acne

Ingredients
- Two teaspoons flaxseeds
- Three teaspoons organic, plain yogurt
- One teaspoon honey

Directions
Soak your flaxseed in hot water. Leave it till the seeds absorb enough water and become more gel-like in consistency. Then proceed to add honey and yogurt to the mix. Apply a thin layer on your face and neck. Massage thoroughly. Leave it for about 15 minutes before rinsing off the mask.

Anti-Acne Lemon Yogurt + Honey Mask

This mask is the perfect remedy for the treatment of acne and clean clog pores. Lemon and milk are an excellent cleanser. Yogurt is also a good softener and cleanser.

Ingredients:
- Two tablespoons of fresh milk
- Two tablespoons of honey
- Fresh juice of one lemon
- One tablespoon of fresh yogurt and lukewarm water

Directions:
Mix all the ingredient thoroughly till it forms a thick consistency. Apply on face and wait for about 2 minutes for it to dry up. Apply the second layer and allow it to dry up. Leave it for 10 minutes, wash off afterwards. This mask should be used three to four times in a week for maximum result.

Cinnamon Honey Mask

Cinnamon is rich in cinnamaldehyde, one of its main constituents, along with eugenol, methyl chavicol, linalool, beta-caryophyllene, and roughage or fiber. The components in cinnamon oil, particularly cinnamaldehyde, eugenol and methyl chavicol have high antimicrobial properties and eliminate microbial infection in acne. While the coarse granules and fiber in cinnamon powder, facilitates exfoliation. This combination of characteristics, along with the benefits of honey makes for an excellent acne treatment.

Ingredient:
- Cinnamon Powder
- Honey

Directions:
make a consistent paste by mixing cinnamon and honey together. Apply the paste on acne affected areas or massage it thoroughly on your face. Leave the paste on your face overnight. Upon waking up the following morning wash off your face with warm water. Repeat this for two weeks to see positive results.
Caution: Many people are allergic to cinnamon, and it can sometimes produce irritation in individuals with unusually sensitive skins. Therefore, this mask should be used after testing somewhere other than the face.

CHAPTER 21

Banana Facial Mask

Recently I was eavesdropping on a conversation between two pretty ladies. Both were sharing their secrets to a radiant look. One of the ladies narrated her special formula on the use of banana as a facial mask. From what I gather from the eavesdropping. Bananas, when combined with other ingredients like baking soda and turmeric, makes for an incredible facial mask.

Well, I have done my research thoroughly on that subject and have come up with a comprehensive banana facial mask remedy. To understand how this works, firstly you have to know that banana is packed with vital vitamins and nutrients like vitamin A, B, E. These vitamin helps fight free radicals and reduce wrinkle. Vitamin A helps get rid of dark spot and blemishes. Vitamin B delays aging, lessens dryness and lightens the skin. Vitamin E helps combats free radical and boost the skin's sun-ray resistance. Potassium gets rid of dry skin by moisturizing and hydrating the cells. When applied as a mask helps smoothen out uneven patches on the face, hydrates the face and fades blemishes. When combined with other ingredients makes the mask even more potent.

Banana, Honey, and Lemon Juice Face Mask

I love this recipe, for what it's worth, I use it myself, and it has this cooling effect on my face. The three ingredients involved are also very potent. Honey has a lightening property which kills bacteria and prevents acne and pimples. Lemon is loaded with citric acid, which lightens dark skin and evens out skin discolouration. What will this mask do for you? Regular application will make your skin brighter and glow. It helps get rid of dark spots.

Ingredient
- One ripe banana
- One teaspoon of honey
- One teaspoon of lemon juice

Directions:
Mash the bananas to make it lump free; I use my fingers to do this. You can use a fork or spoon, whichever way that suits you. Then, add lemon juice and honey to it and mix thoroughly.

How to apply?: Start by rinsing off your face with a mild soap, pat dry with a towel. Using your fingers collect a generous amount and apply on your face. Massage it thoroughly on your face for even distribution. Leave it for about 20 minutes, then rinse off.

Acne-Fighting Banana Face Mask

Trust me this one works well if you want to get rid of pimples. The key ingredients for this acne-fighting banana face mask are turmeric, banana, and baking soda. A friend of mine who is currently battling with acne used this mask recipe and boy it worked. I have written extensively about baking soda in the previous chapter and if you can recall it helps break down dirt, grime, and excess oil, which clogs up your pores. While turmeric has potent antibacterial properties, which destroy bacteria before they can cause pimples. The regular application of this mask will help your skin stay glowing and acne free.

Ingredients:
- 1 small ripe banana
- ½ tsp powdered turmeric
- ½ tsp baking soda

Directions:
Mash your bananas up with your fingers or with the aid of a spoon or fork. Pour in a ½ tablespoon of turmeric powder and ½ tablespoon of baking soda and mix thoroughly together with the mashed bananas.

How to Apply:
Start by washing your face with a mild soap and pat dry. Then, using your fingers, collect a generous amount and apply on face. You will notice a slight sting, it's due to the baking soda, but there is no need to panic. Leave the mask on for about 20 minutes. Wash off with a mild soap, pat dry and add your moisturizer of choice.

Wrinkle Removing Banana Face Mask

This recipe is another great recipe to banish wrinkle. It calls for two more wrinkle busting ingredients that make it a powerful combination. The two add additional ingredients are yogurt and orange juice. Yogurt reduces the appearance of large pores, which makes the skin look aged. While the Vitamin C present in orange helps refreshes skin cells and softens harsh lines and wrinkles.

Ingredients:
- One medium-sized ripe banana
- One tsp orange juice
- One tsp thick yogurt
- Coconut Oil (Optional)

Directions:
Wash your face with a mild soap and pat dry. Mash your bananas with your fingers or fork and add one tablespoon of orange juice and one tablespoon of thick yogurt and mix thoroughly till its lump free. Feel free to add a few drops of coconut oil. Using your fingers, collect the mask and apply to your face and massage till you get an even distribution. You can apply a second coating if you feel that the first wasn't enough. Let it sit for 20 minutes. Now you can wash your face and apply any moisturizer of your choice.

Moisture Locking Banana Mask:

This another fantastic mask recipe on my list that will help you lock in moisture to your skin and keeps your skin looking soft and supple. Avocado has an incredible amount of essential nutrients, including vitamins, minerals and anti-oxidants and is an unusual treatment of wrinkles. Papaya is an excellent source of Vitamin A and

Papain, which helps removes dead skin cells along with breaking down the inactive proteins. It's also have 'Low Sodium Quality', which results in little retention of water. In simple terms it means, it helps you keep your skin hydrated.

Ingredients:
- ½ Papaya
- ½ Banana
- ½ Avocado

Directions:
Combine all the ingredient and mash them all up together till its lump free.

How to apply:
With your fingers collect a reasonable amount and apply to your face. Massage thoroughly on face till it's evenly distributed. Let it sit for about 20 minutes. Wash off with mild soap, pat face dry and moisturize.

CHAPTER 22

13 Herbal Remedies for Glowing Skin

Most women are still trying to uncover the secrets of a glowing skin and many times they spend huge fortune, purchasing chemical driven products. Ending up doing more harm than good. The truth is that for you to have a long-lasting glowing skin that wouldn't pose any problems in the near future, you need to go all natural. A glowing skin only indicates that your skin is healthy. If you wish to go this route, below are 13 herbal remedies for a glowing skin

• Grapes:

To add the much-needed glow to your skin. Cut grapes open and rub the inner part on your face. Leave it for about 15 minutes before washing off.

• Cucumber juice, glycerine and rose water:

Start by mixing cucumber juice, glycerine and rose water together. Apply the mixture on your face. You can leave it on your face while you go about your regular daily routine

• Sandalwood, turmeric, and milk:

Make a paste of sandalwood powder, turmeric powder, and milk. Apply the paste on your face and leave it for about 15 minutes, before washing off with a mild soap. When used often, gives a natural glow and freshness to your face.

• Fresh milk, salt, and lime juice:

This mask works great in cleaning and opening up skin pores. Start by adding a pinch of salt and little lime juice into a reasonable quantity of fresh milk. Apply this mixture on your face and leave it for about 15 minutes. Rinse off afterward.

• Tomato and lemon juice:

This one is so easy that you don't have any reason not to mask. Mix tomato juice with lemon juice. Apply the mixture on your face. Leave it for about 15 minutes before rinsing off. Applying tomato on the face has a cooling effect. This mask will keep your face soft and glowing.

• Turmeric powder, wheat flour, and sesame oil:

This recipe works best in removing unwanted hair on the face. Make a paste of turmeric powder, wheat flour, and sesame oil. Apply the paste on your face. Let it sit for 20 minutes before washing off.

• Cabbage juice and honey:

This recipe will help make your face wrinkle free. Mix cabbage juice with honey and apply it on your face. Leave it for about 15 minutes before rinsing off.

• Carrot juice:

Carrot juice also has a significant role to play in making your skin glow. Extract the juice from carrot using a juicing machine. Apply the juice on your face and leave it for about 15 minutes, before rinsing it off.

• Honey and cinnamon powder

This mask works well in removing pimple on your face. I have used it a couple of times, and it has an amazing way of drying out your pimples overnight. Make a paste of honey and cinnamon powder. Apply the paste on your pimples and leave overnight. Wash off upon waking up.

• Groundnut oil and lime juice:

This mask works with peanut oil and lime juice to prevent the face from pimples, and black head (Original groundnut oil) Mix a little groundnut oil with fresh lime. Apply it on your face and massage thoroughly. Leave for about 15 minutes before rinsing off.

• Aloe Vera juice:

Scoop the gel of aloe vera and apply it on your face. Massage in a circular motion and leave it for about 15 minutes before washing off. Doing this reduces pigments marks while hydrating your skin

• Ghee and glycerine:

Apply a mixture of ghee and glycerine on your face and let it sit for a few minutes. It serves as an excellent moisturizer

• Apricots and yogurt:

Create a paste of apricot and yogurt. Apply the paste on your face and massage thoroughly. Leave it for about 20 minutes before washing off with mild soap. Doing this regularly enhances the skin and gives it a fresh look. If you have a dry skin add honey to the mix.

CHAPTER 23

The Most Effective Remedies for hair Growth

When I set out to write this chapter, I knew that the best person to go to was Mrs. Olivia (my girlfriend's mother). She is one of the African women who believes that the true beauty of every woman lies on her hair. She told me that she has never used any store bought hair care product on her hair.

Judging from the texture of her hair I had no reason to doubt that. Her hair still looks virgin, dark and textured like an ideal Africa woman. One Saturday morning, I placed a call to her, informing her about this remedy book and my plans of including a chapter on natural hair. She was more than delighted to help me.

Onion juice:

On top of her list is the onion remedy, which is a weekly ritual for her hair. Onion contains sulphur which has been proven to boost the production of collagen tissues. These tissues assist in hair growth and sheen.

Directions:

She recommends you start with two to four onions. Grate the onion and squeeze out the juice. If you have a juicer, feel free to use it. Massage the juice on your scalp and leave it on scalp for an hour. Wash off hair and shampoo. You can also dice the onion into pieces and add them into boiling water. Let it simmer for about 5 – 10 minutes, strain and use the water to wash your hair after using a shampoo

Potato Juice

Potatoes are rich in vitamins A, B and C which plays a huge role in hair growth and when deficient by the body can cause hair to be dry and brittle. External application of potato juice on your scalp is beneficial for hair growth too. Simply start by grating or juicing your produce. Massaging the resulting solution on your scalp, leave it to stay for at least 30 minutes before rinsing off. If you have dry hair, she suggests you use potato hair mask instead. For a more rewarding potato mask, she gave me the below recipe

You will need:
- Potatoes – 3
- Egg yolk- from one egg
- Honey – 1 tablespoon

Directions:

She did this particular remedy right in my presence. Start by grating or juicing the potatoes (any method that works for you to extract the juice of potatoes is fine). Add egg yolk and honey to the juice. Mix thoroughly and apply to scalp. Leave it for at least 30 minutes. Then, wash off with mild shampoo and water. She said that the egg yolk and honey lock moisture into the potato juice; which is beneficial for dry hair and helps in growing hair faster.

Eggs White, Olive Oil, and Honey

Everything in our body requires protein to build, the oestrogen hormone responsible for breast development is still composed of protein. Same is also applicable to the hair. That's why she recommend an external application of raw egg to the hair, followed by thorough massaging. Cover with shower cap and let it sit for 30 minutes. To take this even further she gave me the perfect recipe.

You Need:
- Egg white – from 1-2 eggs
- Olive oil- 1 tsp
- Honey- 1tsp

Directions:
Mix egg white, olive oil and honey together in a bowl. Scoop the mixture with your fingers and apply on your scalp. Cover your hair with a shower cap and leave for about 20 minutes. Then wash off with mild shampoo and water

Rinse Hair with Apple Cider Vinegar

If you read the chapter on Apple Cider Vinegar, I need no to say much about the extensive uses of ACV. For what it's worth ACV stimulate the hair follicles, therefore, help them to grow faster. It also aids in maintaining the pH balance of hair, which in turns accelerates hair growth. She recommends you use ACV with water as an after wash rinse. If you don't like the smell of ACV on your hair, pour in a few drops of essential oil like lavender to the mixture before rinsing hair off with it.

Use Fenugreek

The use of Fenugreek as treatment of hair fall is as old as the hills. I will love to call it the wonder herb. Fenugreek contains hormones antecedents that help improve hair growth and strengthens hair follicles. It also contains nicotinic acid and protein that stimulates hair growth. Mrs Olivia loves the fenugreek and coconut milk remedy. Fenugreek, when combined with coconut milk, is one of the best homemade remedies for hair growth

You need:
- Coconut Milk
- Three tablespoons of dried fenugreek seeds

Directions:

Soak two to three tablespoon of fenugreek seeds in water for about 10 hours. Then grind it to make a fine paste. Feel free to mix coconut milk in it. Then apply the paste on your hair and scalp. Leave it to sit for about 30 minutes before washing off with lukewarm water. Alternatively, use the water derived from soaking fenugreek overnight to rinse your hair. Doing this encourages hair growth. She suggests this should be done twice a week.

Ayurvedic Herbs – Indian Gooseberry

Indian gooseberry is another herb she recommends but hardly uses it because of its unavailability. She used it on a few occasions and testified it works. Indian Gooseberry is anti-inflammatory, antioxidant, antibacterial, rich in vitamin C and has exfoliating properties. It also plays a huge role in hair growth. There are so many ways to use this herb for hair growth

- Firstly you can mix one tablespoon of Indian Gooseberry into two tablespoons of coconut oil and heat the mixture. After that strain the oil and massage onto scalp before going to bed. Leave it on hair overnight and shampoo off first thing in the morning

- You can mix two teaspoons each of Indian Goose Berry Powder and lime juice, rub this on your scalp. Leave it overnight and shampoo off the next morning and rinse off with warm water.

- Another way is to mix one-quarter of warm water in a one-half cup of Indian gooseberry powder, let it sit for about 10 minutes. Apply the paste on scalp and massage. Leave it on the scalp for about 15 minutes before rinsing off. This remedy should be followed at least once a week.

CHAPTER 24

Cucumber mask for a fresh and smooth skin

It's was great spending quality time with the whole family – my presence meant a lot to my parents. It's being two years since they last saw me, and am going to make my stay with them worthwhile. Today I managed to convince my mum and sisters that I have a better alternative to their expensive spa treatments.

They were all eager to listen. Because of my reputation as a natural remedy expert, it wasn't hard to convince them after all. Let me get straight to the point here, am going to be using cucumber as my primary ingredient.

Cucumber is not only a rich in water but also contains vast amount of nutrients, antioxidants and have anti-inflammatory properties that's good for your skin.

Cucumber Mask #1

For the 1st recipe, you will need the below ingredients.

- 1 small cucumber
- Vegetable peeler
- Food processor or blender
- 1 tsp. honey (optional)
- 1 tsp. aloe vera gel (optional)
- 1 tbsp. oatmeal
- Coffee grinder
- 1 tbsp. brewer's yeast (optional)

Directions:

Start by peeling your cucumber to get rid of the skin. Then place the cucumber in the blender and blend till it becomes smooth. Add 1tsp of honey or aloe vera into the cucumber puree. This extra ingredients are optional, but they sure do come with their own beauty benefits. The honey has antimicrobial effect while the aloe acts as a moisturizer. The mask needs one more ingredient that will give it an exfoliating effect. So, I choose to use oatmeal. Grind 1 tsp of oat meal into a smooth consistency. I used my coffee grinder. Add the grinded oatmeal into the cucumber puree and mix thoroughly. Finally, add 1 tbsp spoon of brewer's yeast. The yeast is an excellent source of B-complex vitamin which nourishes the skin and tightens pores.

Cucumber Mask #2

This particular one calls for cucumber, mint and egg white. The egg white will help tighten your pores while the cucumber and mint will help hydrate and cleanse your skin.

You need:
- 1 small Cucumber
- Mint
- Egg White from one egg
- Food processor or blender

Directions:

Get your ingredients ready and wash them. Peel the cucumber to get rid of the back, combine all the ingredients together and blend till it forms a smooth consistency. You can now apply on your face. Make sure to leave it for at least for 25 minutes till it dries up. Rinse off afterward and pat dry

Cucumber Mask #3

This third mask is packed with rich anti-oxidant which helps rid your face of wrinkles and fine lines. Cucumber, on the other hand, is an excellent source of silica which helps improve your complexion and health of your skin. Due to its high water content it hydrates and makes your skin glow.

You will need:
- 1 small Cucumber
- Aloe vera
- ½ Lemon
- Food processor or blender

Directions:

Get all your ingredients ready. Squeeze out the juice from the lemon. But you will only be using 1 tsp of lemon juice to prevent it from burning your face. Then scrape the gel from the aloe vera leaf and keep it aside. Now, peel your cucumber – put all the produce into a blender and blend till it forms a thick consistency. Please, this mask should not be applied on sensitive parts like the mouth and eyes.

Cucumber Mask #4

The fourth mask calls for cucumber, brown sugar, honey, and milk. Your guess is right, the brown sugar acts as an exfoliant. Boy, when you are done using this mask your face will feel fresh rejuvenated.

You need:
- 1 Small Cucumber
- 1 tsp Brown Sugar
- 1 tsp Honey
- ¼ cup Milk
- Food processor or blender

Directions:

Get all your ingredients together. Peel the cucumber to get the green back away. Blend the cucumber to a smooth consistency. Add 1 tsp of honey, ¼ cup of milk and 1 tsp of brown sugar and mix thoroughly. You can add it back to the blender to make the solution blend properly. Apply the mask on your face and leave for about 20 minutes to dry up. Then wash off the mask.

Cucumber Mask #5

The fifth mask recipe calls for yogurt and cucumber. Yogurt contains lactic acid, an alpha hydroxy acid, both of which helps get rid of dead skin cells. The yogurt combined with cucumber will help soothe sunburned skin. If you have discolored and uneven skin tone, I suggest you try out this mask. It's also great for pimples.

You need:
- 1 Small Cucumber
- 1 tsp Yogurt
- Food processor or blender

Directions:

Get all your ingredients ready. Make sure you are using plain unsweetened and unflavored yogurt to avoid skin irritations. Peel the cucumber and blend it together with the yogurt. If you have dry skin add a bit of coconut or olive oil. Apply on face and leave for about 20 minutes, let it dry before washing off.

Cucumber Mask #6

The sixth cucumber mask is like the first one but with exclusion of oatmeal. The presence of honey in this recipe helps promote the growth of new tissues while contributing to a healthy and supple skin.
Honey is naturally antibacterial, so it's great for acne treatment and prevention. It is rich in antioxidant that helps slow down aging process.

You need:
- 1 tsp Honey
- 1 small Cucumber
- 1 tsp Aloe Vera
- Food processor or blender

Directions:
Peel the cucumber and blend with your blender. Add 1 tsp of honey into the blender. Keep blending till it forms a smooth consistency. Apply to your face and massage on face properly. Leave it for 15 minutes before drying off. Rinse off and pat dry.

Natural Beauty tips when using Cucumber Face Masks

If you are using your cucumber right out from the refrigerator. Please let it reach room temperature before using it for your mask

- I have learnt to put an apron or place an old cloth on my body while applying the mask, to avoid the mask dripping on my cloth.

- Before applying the mask, wash your face thoroughly. If you wear makeups – I need not to tell you that you have to cleanse and wash your face first.

- To make the mask more effective, do a hot water steam, this will open your pores, while making the mask effective.

- While waiting for the cucumber mask to dry. You can place two slices of cucumber on your eyes. Doing this helps reduce puffiness and diminish dark circle around your eyes

- Use rose water to cleanse your face after washing off the mask, this will help close your pores and re-fresh your skin.

- Don't be too eager to throw away the excess mask, you can still use it for your neck, chest and shoulder. It can also be stored in the refrigerator for future use – but don't store for too long.

- When you are done with your mask – consider applying a moisturizing gel or lotion of your choice.

CHAPTER 25

Effective Ways to tighten Loose Vagina

Loose vagina has become a huge problem for both men and women. It places a huge demand on men. That explains why most men with average size penis seek an alternative remedy to enlarge their penis. The truth is that it's difficult to satisfy a lady with a loose vagina.

Factors like giving birth can cause a loose vagina. During labor the virginal and cervical muscles contract and repeatedly expand, coupled with the arrival of the baby through the vaginal opening. These activities may damage the tissues, muscles and perineum around the vagina. Although the damage can be healed within a few weeks after delivery. It certainly wouldn't make the vagina as it was, prior delivery. The significant drop in the estrogen or hormone either due to episiotomy during childbirth, lactation and the side effects of oral contraceptives can lead to a loose vaginal.

The simple truth is that before you can regain a tight vagina and maintain it elasticity after delivery, your estrogen level has to be high. But it unfortunate that most mothers experience a significant drop in their estrogen level after birth and during lactation. The use of oral contraceptive can also worsen the condition.

Although your doctor will advise you to do Kegels to strengthen your virginal muscles, the truth is that the only way to restore your vaginal walls is through sufficient supply of woman's estrogen to their genital organs.

The key to increasing the estrogen level is the supply of Phytoestrogens, which are plant-derived xenoestrogens, not generated within the endocrine system but by consuming phytoestrogen plants. Unlike synthetic estrogen, phytoestrogen is considered to be a safer alternative, because it mimics human estrogen. Several studies have shown that it helps lower the risk of osteoporosis, heart disease, breast cancer, and menopausal symptoms.

There are many phytoestrogen sources out there. If you read the chapter on breast enlargement, which I listed a few like fenugreek.

When the case is tightening, and rejuvenation, Pueraria mirifica, Oak gall and Witch Hazel has shown aggressive results with estrogenic activities in stimulating collagen and elastin production, while increasing the fiber muscle mass.

These herbs can also be used to remedy vaginal dryness, itching, soreness and white discharge.

You might be wondering, how do I know if my vagina is loose or not?

- The simple test I recommend is to slide your forefinger (the finger close to the thumb) into your vagina and clasp it with the labia by contracting the muscles. Then insert your index and middle fingers to assess tightness as compared to a single finger. If you can add your ring, middle, and index finger hold together and cannot feel anything, then it is most likely that you're loose.

- Also, if you are the type that masturbates and finds it necessary to insert a large object to achieve sexual stimulation, then you might have a loose vagina. Also most women with loose vagina experience urine leakage commonly known as stress incontinence. Another sign of loose vagina is having difficulties achieving orgasm. There is no need to panic. The truth is that as women grow old, they may start to complain about a loose vagina.

Pueraria Mirifica

Pueraria Mirifica is well used in Thailand for medical purposes, mainly for female growth hormone supplementation. It is found in the wild, Myanmar and Northeastern Thailand and also known as Kwao Krua. Pueraria Mirifica has been shown to increase sex drive, increase vaginal moisture, the thickness of vaginal walls and increase breast size and also reduce the appearance of stretch marks. Further studies have shown that the estrogenic activities in Pueraria Mirifica are more active than that in fenugreek and black cohosh. A study from Mahidol University, Thailand, revealed that, the estrogenic activities of P. Mirifica extract occurred significantly in the vaginal and urethral epithelium with certain doses (100 and 1,000 mg/kg/day). Which means, their estrogenic activities are clinically proven and have an ability in regenerating vaginal tissues. Therefore, those who want to rejuvenate their vaginal wall or tissues, the estrogeninc activities from these phytoestrogens is highly recommended. Pueraria is available in the form of capsules, liquid or powder. It can also be applied topically. For the best results, you should take this supplement along with a food or beverage that is high in calcium, such as milk, cheese, sesame seeds or almonds, as it seems calcium helps increase the absorption of phytoestrogens, which are the main active ingredients in Pueraria and many other herbs. Another studies archived about Menopause on October 2007 also revealed that, "the phytoestrogen from this plant showed an ability to rejuvenate vaginal tissues, overcome vaginal dryness from the root cause (estrogen deficiency), enhance vaginal fluid production, and atrophy vaginal epithelium in healthy postmenopausal women.

Oak Gall

Oak Gall also known as masikai in Tamil and manjakani in Malaysia is a favorite herb, more especially in Tamil Nadu. In Asian and Mid-Eastern countries this herb is well used in restoring vaginal tightness. The extract of this plant is very rich in Tannin and phytoestrogens and is capable of tightening the vaginal tissues instantly. Also, it is also rich in phytochemical substances. With various health benefits like (anti-fungi, anti-bacterial, anti-viral, anti-inflammatory, anti-diabetics, and local anesthetic), such as gallic acids, ellagic acid, piperonylic acid ester, antioxidants, calcium, fiber, vitamin A and C, iron, carbohydrates, and some other proteins. This plant doesn't just stop at tighten up and rejuvenating the virginal muscle and walls, but can also help in enhancing sexual and physical performance, maintain healthy uterus, improves bowel movement, stabilizes the pH levels and reduces excessive vaginal fluids. Due to its large properties, it is widely found as an active ingredient in most cosmetic products that deals with vaginal tightening.

Kegel Exercise

The kegel exercise helps tighten the vagina. It strengthens the pelvic floor muscles that surround the vagina. Kegel exercise involves a woman contracting the muscles of her groin and then relaxing them after 10 seconds. Most people are confused on how to locate their pelvic muscle. To find your pelvic muscle try this: while urinating stop in midstream and hold for a while and continue. Try this at intervals till you finish urinating. If you succeed you've got the right muscles. Another way to do kegels is by tighten your pelvic floor muscles, hold the contraction for about five minutes, then relax for five seconds. Try doing this for at least four or five times in a row, gradually work up to keep the muscles contracted for about 10 seconds at a time and relaxing for 10 seconds between contractions. While doing Kegels, make sure to tightening only your pelvic floor muscles and not the muscles in your abdomen, thighs or buttocks. Lastly do not hold your breath while doing this, breathe freely.

Vaginal Cone

Vaginal cones are small weight which you can place in your vagina to help train your pelvic floor muscles. A 1995 study by Norwegian scientists shows that the cone helps increase muscle tone. Whether the women involved where able to retain the cone or not. The study also showed improved coordination of pelvic floor muscle activity. To use the cone properly, start by inserting the cone with the appropriate weight and use your pelvic muscle to keep the cone in place. Start with the cone you can hold for one minute and do this twice a day. Then gradually you can increase the length of time you can hold the cone. Do this till you can hold the cone for about 15 minutes twice daily.

Ben-wa balls

As strange as the name sound, it's still one of the best tools for an amazing sex life. Ben-wa balls helps strengthen your muscles to stop or hold urine flow, which is good for older women who are beginning to lose urinary control. It also causes clitoral erection during sexual arousal and rhythmically contraction during sexual arousal. It also supports the bladder, uterus and rectum. Ben-wa balls are made of two hollow brass balls, of which one was empty with the other containing either mercury or a smaller heavy metal balls. The empty ball should be inserted inside the cervix, then followed by the 2nd "loaded" ball until they make contact with each other. When the balls are properly in place, even the slightest movement of your hips will cause the balls to move, therefore producing a pleasant vibration.

Kegels should also be performed to help hold them in and to strengthen the pelvic floor muscles, while improving the vagina's elasticity.

* ***Directions:***

Start by lubricating the balls and then gently slide it into your vagina, while in a relaxed position. Hold the balls inside your vagina, by tensing your leg muscles together and doing kegel exercise. Now you can sit up and keep them in while moving around the house

Leg Raise

Leg raise is one of the simple exercise that can help strengthen your pelvic muscle. To do this exercise, lie down on your back and lift your legs upwards one after the other without bending any of them. I recommend you do this exercise about 10 minutes and repeat at least twice daily for best benefits.

Lastly, if you are having sex and looking for a quick and easy trick to create a feeling of a tight vagina, have the man on top position. As soon as he inserts his penis, he should lift himself up a bit, while you close your legs, with your thighs squeezing the penis. This simple technique will increase the sensation and help you enjoy the ride.

CHAPTER 26

Ways to enlarge your breast naturally

For most women breast enlarging their breast have become a pressing issue. Some are willing to go any length to add an extra inch to their breast. While some with deep pockets chose to embark on the fat-graft mammoplasty approaches used to increase the breast size, change the shape and also alter the texture.

It might interest you to know that you don't need to go under the knife to enlarge your breast. I have taken the required time to research on the natural alternatives for breast enlargement. Although you shouldn't expect drastic result with this as that of Breast Augmentation. But you should be able to see a subtle increase in your breast size.

Fenugreek

Fenugreek long had a history of enlarging the breast. It also contains diosgenin which is used in making synthetic estrogen. You might be wondering what the hell is estrogen? In lay terms, when a woman is in her puberty, she produces estrogens naturally. Estrogen helps in the development of new tissues. This hormone determines the size, shape and fullness of the woman's breast. If the estrogen level is low, this might result to smaller, less developed breast. Fenugreek helps promote the growth of new breast cells while increasing the size and fullness of the breast. It does this by mimicking the effects of estrogen and stimulating the production of prolactin. These are the major hormones crucial to the development of the breast. It might also interest you to know that among all the herbs used for breast enlargement, fenugreek has the highest concentration of the useful plant compounds, and it's considered the finest herb for enhancing the feminine beauty. Also, it aids in sexual stimulation, balances blood sugar levels, and contain choline which helps thinking process.

How to use fenugreek for breast enlargement

- **Use Fenugreek Paste**

This remedy was gotten from my grandmother's journal, although I fine-tuned it a bit, it's pretty much the same.

You need:
- Two tablespoons of olive oil
- Ten tablespoons of fenugreek seeds
- Four teaspoons of saw palmetto (Very potent for breast enlargement)

This recipe calls for saw palmetto and fenugreek because they both contain estrogen that will mimic the real estrogen in your body. Roast and dry your fenugreek seeds. Grind the dried seed to a powdery consistency. Add your saw palmetto and a reasonable amount of olive oil. The principal purpose of adding the olive oil to the mixture is to extract the active ingredient in the saw palmetto and fenugreek. Mix thoroughly till you get a consistent paste with no lumps.

Take a reasonable amount of the paste and massage on your beast. Leave it for about one to two hours on your breast before rinsing off. After your massage, set your heating pad to a low or medium heat and apply it to your breast for about 15 – 20 minutes. The warmth boosts circulation to your breast and helps your body absorb more of the herb.

Alternatively, consuming at least one teaspoon of ground fenugreek seeds and a half teaspoon of ground saw palmetto daily, can have the same effect. Doing this wouldn't only increase your breast but add an ample amount of antioxidant and loads of minerals and vitamins to your body. But be warned this might give you slight dizziness, stomach pain, diarrhea, lactation, smelly armpits and vomiting if you consume more than the required amount. Moderation is the key here. Also bear in mind that this remedy will not give that massive boob's but will add millimeters to a centimeter's enlargement to your breast.

Another excellent solution to consider is fennel seed and fenugreek. The remedy can be used as a paste or taken orally as described with the fenugreek and saw palmetto treatment. Fennel seeds are also known to increase the number of fluids in the breast tissues which are ideal for adding firmness to the breast while expanding the size dramatically.

Breast Massage

Breast massage is another effective way to increase the size of your breast. Since the hormone estrogen flows through the blood stream. Massaging the breast can help improve blood flow, which in turns causes more estrogen to reach the breast receptors and stimulates breast growth. Also, the hormone prolactin is released when breast tissues or the nipple are stimulated. This hormone also helps with breast enlargement.

To perform a breast massage at home, I suggest you try out the Chi breast massage, which is the most efficient and accessible breast massage techniques. The chi breast massage technique works with your pressure points to help with the flow of chi energy around your breast. It also helps improve circulation and increase prolactin flow in your breast.

- *Directions:*
Place your hands over your breast with the fingers open slightly, covering as much area of your breast as possible. Put your right hand on your right breast and your left hand on your left breast. Press down firmly and move your hands in an inward rotating circle. Be sure to move the breast tissue themselves as opposed just sliding the fingers across the skin. Rotate both breasts simultaneously from 180 to 360 rotation. Repeat this twice daily for fast results. Other massaging techniques you should know are Reiki Massage, Feng Shui Breast Massage, Lymph Draining Massage, and Breast Slapping Technique.

Skin Brushing or Fat Transfer Massage.

This breast massage serves the purpose of reducing the belly fat and increasing the fat in your chest. Start by applying few drops of coconut oil on your palms. Then rub your palms together for a while to produce heat. Sweep the fat from your waist and upper arm and gradually move it up to your breasts.

Exercise

Exercise help you increase your burst size. But particular types of workout targets the breast region correctly. These types of exercises help in building up the pectoral muscles, as well as the glandular and fat tissues in your breast. When these exercises are done regularly, it makes your breast larger and toned
- Push Ups
- Wall Push-ups
- Dumbbells Flys
- Reverse Dumbbells Flys
- Chest Dips
- Elevated push ups

Am not going to go into further details about these exercises on this book but Feel free to research on these exercise with your spare time

Amino Acids

Growth homes are critical for breast growth. But the sad truth is that growth homes start to drop at the age of 25. Not to worry much, there is a way around this. Since hormone is protein, it makes much sense that adding certain amino acid to your system can boost growth hormones, which in turns helps with breast growth. If you are confused on which amino acid to use, I suggest you try arginine, glutamine, and lysine. These amino acids help increase the hormone by 300%. You will also benefit from the added advantage of slow aging and burning of fat.

Vitamins

Vitamins work very much like breast augmentation. Some women choose to go this route, which I think it's a better alternative because it helps increase breast size for little cost, unlike breast augmentation. Vitamin A, C, and E are the three vitamins that help with breast enlargement and healthy skin. Vitamin C produces collagen which is essential for keeping the skin toned and firm (helps the breast stay perky). Vitamin A is responsible for keeping the skin nourished while Vitamin

E helps in your overall health and healthy skin production.

Herbs

Herbal supplement like saw palmetto, dong quai, damiana, and wild yam can contribute to the enlargement of the breast. Taking saw palmetto supplement will help increase the size of the mammary glands, am sure of this, because several women have testified to this. You will even get the added advantage of healthy urinary system function and smooth digestion and a healthy appetite.

Pueraria Mirifica

Pueraria Mirifica has been used in Thailand for medicinal purposes for many years, mainly as a female hormone supplement. Pueraria Mirifica is a plant found in the wild in Myanmar and Northeastern Thailand. It is also known as kwao krua.

Women who are looking for an alternative to breast augmentation often turn to Pueraria Mirifica. One study has suggested that 70 percent of women who use Pueraria Mirifica noticed an increase in their breast size. Not only does it increase breast size, but it can also reduce the appearance of stretch marks.

Pueraria is widely available in the form of a capsule, liquid or powder. It can also be applied topically. For best results, you should take this supplement along with foods or beverages that are high in calcium, such as milk, cheese, sesame seeds or almonds. Because calcium helps increase the absorption of phytoestrogens, which are the main active ingredients in Pueraria and many other herbs.

Saw palmetto

Saw palmetto is available in capsule, tablet and tea form. I recommend you drink two to three cups of saw palmetto tea every day or take the supplements twice daily. I suggest you check with your doctor to verify if Saw Palmetto pills are safe for you.

Dong quai

Dong quai supplement will assist in improving circulation throughout the body and to the breast while adding in breast enlargement and balancing hormones. It produces the hormones progesterone which plays a vital role in breast development. The usual recommended dose is to take a capsule three times a day to see visible result.

Wild yam

Wild yam will stimulate hormone production which aids in breast enlargement. It contains a natural progesterone from its fat called diosgenin, which has a similar molecular structure as the human progesterone. This hormone plays the role of balancing estrogen level in your body. When it enters and stays in your breast in a huge amount, it stimulates fat tissues to increase in size, roundness, and fullness. It is also used as an aphrodisiac, for the treatment of impotence in men - and for inhibiting sexual desire in women. This herb is suggested to be taken one capsule of about 300 mg three times a day for faster results.

Damiana

Damiana helps improve mammary gland development, which aids in increasing breast size.

Fennel Seeds

Fennel Seeds contain flavonoids, which have estrogenic properties. They assist in the growth of breast tissues in non-nursing mothers and boost breast milk quantity in nursing mothers. Fennel is also used to treat amenorrhea, angina, asthma, heartburn, high blood pressure and to increase sexual desire in women. It's recommended you take about one capsule three times a day for it to take effect.

Red Clover:

Red Clover contains four phytoestrogen which includes the presence of genistein component. These phytoestrogens like genistein are critical in breast growth, as it helps bind receptors, responsible and strictly associated with breast development. It combines well with other traditional anti-cancer herbs, turmeric and ginger root, and also combines well with your femle hormone balance and natural breast health and enhancement programs. It's recommended you take this herb one capsule three times daily. Alternatively, you can add one or two teaspoons of dried red clover flowers to one cup of hot water. Allow it to steep for 30 minutes. Then strain and drink this tea two or three times a day. Follow this remedy for a few months to get the desired result.

CHAPTER 27

Treat Hair loss with these Herbal Remedies

Balding is not a threatening condition, so there is virtually no reason to panic. The condition is sometimes called androgenetic alopecia. It certainly doesn't look bad on all guys. Jason Statham is a great example of a guy rocking his balding. Most male folks will do anything to remedy this situation.

I once knew a man who spent a fortune on expensive treatments to for baldness. The point here is that if you are cool with your balding, and it doesn't make you feel less confident, then, there is no reason to go the extra mile. But if you have concerns about it, why not try out a few home remedies. Men are more likely to go bald than women. In men, it usually takes 15-25 years to go bald. In this piece, I tried my best to outline the most efficient remedies for balding. They are simple ingredients you can quickly source and you wouldn't break the bank buying a few of them.

Fenugreek seed for Balding

While in India, I meet several Ayurvedic Doctors and I learned a lot about Fenugreek. Fenugreek is of the most used ingredient for baldness. The seeds are an excellent source of nicotinic acid and protein, which helps strengthen and rebuilding hair shafts. They are rich in hormones that help restore hair growth. To use fenugreek in this fashion, grind 1 – 3 tablespoon of fenugreek and add a little water to form a paste. Apply the resulting paste on your head and leave it for about an hour. Wash off with water. Repeat this twice a week for best results.

Henna for Balding

Henna is mostly used to dye skin, hair, and fingernails. As well as fabrics including silk, wool, and leather. Henna is also used for hair conditioning. When mixed with mustard, henna can remedy baldness

Get this:
- 100 gm Henna leaves
- 250 gm Mustard oil

Directions:
Pour the mustard oil into a sauce pan and add henna leaves – let it boil for a while and bring it to cool down. Strain the resulting mixture and store in a tight jar. You can now massage it on your scalp. Do this every day.

Camphor oil for Balding

These days we go through a whole lot of stress. From work stress to family stress. A whole lot unending vicious circle of stress and anxiety. This can sometimes lead to hair loss. When this is the case, camphor oil is the best remedy to avert hair loss Camphor is an excellent relaxant and can help relieve you from stress and nervous tension – while helping you calm down. It enhances blood flow to your scalp and hair re-growth. Camphor oil can work well with any hair oil, but I suggest you use coconut oil. Work it up your scalp and massage on bald patches. When this is done on daily basis, you should begin to see improvements.

Lemon Seeds and Peppercorns for Balding

I heard about this from a herbalist friend of mine – she claims it worked for most of her clients. She told me that this remedy helps increase blood circulation to the scalp and can help for a rapid hair growth.

Get this:
- Seven lemon seeds
- Ten black peppercorns

Directions:
- Crush the seed of lemon and peppercorn together.
- Apply the resulting paste on the bald patches.
- Leave thus for about 10 – 15 minutes.
- Add lemon juice if the paste feels dry.
- This might cause you a little itchiness and irritation, but do not panic. It's normal for this remedy. For quick results apply this treatment twice daily for a week.

Onion for Balding

When the onion remedy broke out newly on the internet with claims of improving hair growth, I quickly gave it a try, and it turned out that the claims might be true. Onions help cleanse the scalp and hair follicles while still promoting thicker hair. This is due to its capacity to produce catalase. Onion is also useful in averting gray hair. To use onion for hair loss, Start by peeling off the outer part. Using a juicer, juice the onion to extract the liquid content. If you are using a blender, filter out the liquid using a kitchen strainer or a washcloth. Gently apply the resulting onion juice on your scalp and massage for about 10 minutes. Wash off with water. Beware, this will make your hair stink, but the benefits are worth more than the smell. Follow up by washing off hair with a mild shampoo.

Honey and Onion for Balding

Onion also forms a potent mix with honey and helps get rid of balding. Mix the onion juice with honey and massage on scalp. If you can't juice the onion, Cut into half and rub it on the bald area, followed by honey. Wash off hair with a mild shampoo afterward.

Aloe Vera for Hairloss

Aloe vera has also shown to be capable in this department. It is known to contain enzymes that helps open clogged hair follicles while averting hair fall. It is also a rich source of vitamin and minerals which promote hair growth.

Ingredients:
- Aloe vera
- Lukewarm water

Directions:
- Scrape out the gel from aloe vera leaf and apply the gel on your scalp.
- Massage on scalp for a few minutes.
- Leave it for a few hours and rinse off with lukewarm water.
- You can do this four times weekly.
- You can also combine aloe vera with honey, which makes another potent mix.

Saw Palmetto for Balding

I have always known saw palmetto be an excellent herb used in the treatment of a variety of ailments such as urinary tract infection, testicular inflammation, cough and respiratory congestion. It has also made its name as a breast enlargement herb – and also helps in hair restoration, prostate health, sexual vigor and nutritive tonic. It blocks an enzyme responsible for converting hormone testosterone into dihydrotestosterone which leads to androgenic alopecia. People on blood thinners or individuals who are hemophiliac should avoid having saw palmetto herb. Saw palmetto comes in several different forms, which are: whole dried berries, tablets, liquid extracts and powdered capsules. Tablets and capsules are easiest to find and are the only forms that have been investigated by researchers.

Castor Oil for Balding

Castor oil can be used to improve blood circulation to the hair follicles while nourishing hair roots and making your hair stronger and longer. Castor oil is an excellent source of vitamin E, protein and has antibacterial, anti-fungal and anti-inflammatory which helps clear infections related to skin and scalp problems. Make sure to use only unrefined castor oil, because it contains more nutrients and healing properties. Since castor oil has so much viscosity. It makes perfect sense to mix it with a carrier oil like olive oil, coconut oil, almond oil or jojoba oil.

You need:
- Castor oil
- Plastic cap
- Shampoo

Directions:
Place the castor oil over medium heat and let it heat up for a while. Bring it down and let it cool a little. Apply on scalp and massage for a few minutes. Let is stay overnight. Cover with a shower cap. In the morning upon waking up wash off

with shampoo. Alternatively, mix almond oil with castor oil to form a smooth and fragrant oil. Almond is a rich source of vitamin E, which strengthens the hair strand and follicles. Mix equal amount of castor and almond oil. Apply this mixture to the scalp and repeat the process mentioned above.

Hibiscus for Balding

Hibiscus is one of the best-known herbs for hair and popular for promoting hair growth. It's well active in regenerating hair in bald patches and averting hair fall. It is also used in preventing premature graying of hair. You can either use the tea of dried hibiscus petal or make your concoction.

You need:
- Hibiscus flowers
- Coconut oil
- Curry leaves
- Gooseberry (amla)

Directions:
Combine all ingredient in a bowl and bring it to boil. Bring it down from heat and allow it to cool down. Strain the oil and massage it on hair. Leave it for 30 minutes before washing off. Do this daily for best result. If you can't gather all the above ingredients. Simply, boil hibiscus in water and mix it with lime juice. Apply the resulting mixture to your bald patches. Leave it for a period before washing off with water.

Olive Oil for Baldness

Olive oil plays a vital role in hair growth, and it's widely used to enhance hair growth on areas where bald patches occur. It can also be employed by both men and women to combat hair loss and strengthen hair.

Ingredients:
- One tsp Olive oil
- One tsp Cinnamon powder
- One tsp of Honey
- Mild shampoo
- Microwave safe bowl or pan

Directions:
Pour the one tsp of olive oil into a saucepan and place it on a stove, you can use a microwave. The aim is to warm up the olive oil a bit. Now, add honey and cinnamon powder into the olive oil. Stir it thoroughly and apply on scalp. Let it sit about

20 minutes. Wash it off afterward with a mild shampoo, followed by water. Do this three times a week for best results. Alternatively, olive oil can be combined with cumin seeds and rubbed on the bald patches. While using, these treatments endeavor to massage the oil into your scalp every night and leave till day break. When doing this don't forget to place a protective cover on your pillow, to prevent it from getting oily. Shampoo out first thing the next morning.

CHAPTER 28

Effective Home Remedies for Wrinkles

A particular woman came to me complaining about how she couldn't seem to get rid of her wrinkle after breaking her bank to buy an expensive beauty product, which ended up doing her more harm than good. Looking at her face, I could clearly see what seems to look like a map of Africa on her face. Which was as a result of the adverse effect caused by this product. Now she's not only battling with her wrinkles but also battling with the scars the product left on her face.

This event brought me to this subject of wrinkles and how to remedy it. Wrinkles only form when the skin thins and loses its elasticity. Wrinkles occur as a natural part of aging process, which is as a result of the weakening and breakdown of the collagen and elastin in the connective tissue of the skin, due to the changes in fibroblast that produce collagen and elastin. No matter what you do, you will develop wrinkles if you live long enough. The first sign of wrinkles is usually around the eyes – smile lines or "crow's feet." Followed by the check and lips. Other factors also help determine the rate and the extent of wrinkles. These factors include diet, nutrition, muscle tone, habitual facial expression, stress, lack of proper skin care, exposure to environmental pollutant and lifestyle habits such as smoking. But do you know what I found out lately? Exposure to the sun play a huge role on wrinkle appearing on your face – in fact, the sun is your worst enemy. It dries out your skin and also leads to the generation of free radicals that can damage skin cells. The ultraviolet rays from the sun erode the elastic tissues in the skin causing wrinkle to appear.

• Diet Remedies for Wrinkles:

Most times what you get into your body can significantly influence the look and feel of your skin. It might also interest you to know that the food you eat plays a greater role on how fresh or supple your skin looks.

• Drink plenty of Water

Most people only drink water when they are thirsty, if you are like this, I must tell you that you are going about it the wrong way. It's imperative you drink at least 2 quarts of water even when you don't feel thirsty. Doing this helps keep the skin hydrated and flush away toxins while discouraging the formation of wrinkles.

• Have foods with wrinkle fighting elements

Fatty acid should be obtained from cold-pressed vegetable oils. Saturated, and animal fats should be avoided. Also, food rich in omega-3 fatty acids, trace retinol, iron, vitamin E and C and mono-unsaturated fat should be encouraged. These foods includes:
- Tomatoes
- Berries
- Green Tea
- Yogurt and Kefir
- Avocados
- Dark colored fruits and vegetables
- Nuts like almonds, walnuts
- Legumes, beans, and lentils

- Eggs
- Liver
- Oily fish like tuna, salmon, herring and sardines
- Flaxseed and sunflower seeds and oil.
- Brazil nuts
- Whole grains like brown rice, whole wheat, and oats.
- Shellfish
- Green and white tea
- Soy foods (you should have them in moderation only)

Including all these foods in your daily diet will sure keep the wrinkles away.

• Lifestyle Remedies for Wrinkles

Unhealthy lifestyle choices can significantly lead to the early development of wrinkles. So before you complain about wrinkles ask yourself, is your lifestyle healthy? You can't smoke heavily and expect to stay wrinkle free.

Below are some unhealthy choices we make that leads to the early stage of wrinkles development.

• Sleep sufficient and sleep right:

According to what I read on prevention.com – Estée Lauder, a cosmetics company teamed up with UH Case Medical Center to evaluate how sleep—or lack thereof—affected the skin of 60 women. It turns out that, those who slept only 5 hours every night for a month had twice as many wrinkles and spots compared to those who slept for 7 hours. They also recovered from sunburn significantly slower than those who clocked in more zzz's. These findings were presented in May at the International Investigative Dermatology meeting in Edinburgh, Scotland. This shows that at night, energy and cellular functions focus more on repair and recovery to prepare the skin defensive mechanism against the environment the next morning. Which goes to imply that less sleep translate to less repair, thereby causing wrinkles over time.

• Don't Stress:

I know of a colleague at the office, who stressed herself more than necessary. I was shocked when I found out that she was just 22, but the wrinkles on her face made her look 35. A particular study was conducted in 2004 to show the link between chronic stress and aging. This study revealed that the telomeres (structures at the ends of chromosomes that shorten with aging) also shorten prematurely in people experiencing long-term psychological stress, in effect, prematurely "aging" the cells.

Personally, I believe that anything that gives you much stress is not worth it at all. If you job puts you into lots of pressure, It's time to get another job. I suggest you indulge yourself in work you love, follow your passion (if you have one), develop a hobby, read books, swim, do yoga, spend time with your spouse and children. Whatever it is that will take the stress away do for your peace of mine.

• Avoid smoking, alcohol and caffeine

Smoking can significantly lead to wrinkles. It dries out the skin by upsetting the body's mechanism for renewing the skin. Dermatologist says that long-term smoking can result in premature aging. Researchers suspected that smoking disrupted the body's natural process of breaking down the old skin and renewing it.

• Protect and preserve yourself from wrinkle forming sources

You don't have control over the natural aging process – but there are certain things you can do to prevent wrinkle appearing on your face prematurely.

• Protect skin from harmful sun-rays

Since ultraviolet ray from the sun can damage your skin collagen leading to wrinkles. The best advice I can give to you is to stay away from direct exposure to sunlight. If your job entails you stay under the sun, resign. If you must go under the sun, wear a sunscreen with an SPF of at least 15 whenever going out under the sun, which is effective in protecting your skin against UVA and UVB radiation from the sun. I also recommend you go for enhance sunscreen containing vitamin E or soy isoflavones, which shields and strengthens your skin by assisting the reproducing collagen. Strong sunrays can make you squint therefore leading to wrinkle formation around your eyes, so it pays to invest in good quality sunglasses – cheaper brands can damage your eyes. If you love hats, you are at an advantage here, and if you can use the umbrella under the sun without feeling embarrassed, good. Anything that keeps you away from direct sun-light is ok.

• Use cosmetics with care

If you read this piece from the beginning, and you remember what I wrote about my encounter with a certain woman who damaged her skin with over the counter skin care product. It saddens me that most of us still fall prey to these companies. We often break our banks to buy things that are unhealthy and damaging to our skin. If you must buy these products, try as much as possible to avoid the ones with alcohol in them. For instance, alcohol based toning products should be avoided.

Instead, use witch hazel or herbal/floral water. Use coconut oil often to moisturize your skin; a skin lacking moisture tends to wrinkle fast. Avoid the use of concealer to hide wrinkles. Trust me they often make your wrinkles more prominent by settling themselves in the spaces in between your fine lines.

• Powerful home Remedies for Wrinkles

I think I have said more than enough on the dos and don'ts of wrinkles. It's time to dive straight into the actual home remedies to prevent wrinkles – which is the main purpose of this piece.

• Avocado Mask

Avocado is a rich source of vitamin E and monounsaturated fat – loaded with anti-aging elements. Avocado fruit is packed with anti-aging elements. Avocado is often used to get rid of wrinkles.

You will need:
- ½ Avocado
- 2 tsp Fresh cream
- 2 tsp of Flaxseeds
- 1 tsp of Honey

Directions:
In a medium size bowl combine mashed avocado, flaxseed powder, fresh cream, and honey. Mix all together to form a paste. Apply the paste on your face or other parts with wrinkles. Leave it for an hour before washing off with lukewarm water. This mask serves as an excellent moisturizes for your skin. When used regularly, you will see amazing results.

• Papaya-Banana Mask

Papaya and Banana are a force to reckon with if the case is beauty remedies. You will see these two ingredients in virtually every beauty treatments. Banana is loaded with beneficial nutrients that help in producing new skin cells, which helps getting rid of the old sagging skin. While Papaya, on the other hand, contains certain enzymes that remove your dead skin cells to give place to new once.

You will need:
- Papaya
- Banana

Directions:
Mash both papaya pieces and banana together and mix thoroughly. Apply on your skin and leave for 20 minutes. Then wash off with lukewarm water.

Egg White Wonder

Egg white are mostly used to tighten and refine pores. It contains essential nutrients and vitamins. Simply whip up the white of an egg and apply it to your face as a mask. Rinse off after 20 minutes. Below is a simple DIY egg mast recipe

You will need:
- Egg white- from one egg
- 1 tsp Honey
- 1 tsp Milk
- Avocado/Olive/Coconut or any other oil- few drops

Directions:
Mix all the ingredient together and apply on your face. Leave it for about 20 minutes before rinsing off with warm water

Honey

Honey does wonders on the skin, it's perhaps the most ancient remedy used for beautiful skin and highly effective when it comes to wrinkles. Applying honey on your face and washing it off after 20 minutes can make a great difference in your skin. Below is a simple honey remedy for wrinkles

You will need:
- 4 tsp of Milk powder
- 2 tablespoon of Honey
- Warm water
- A small towel

Directions:
Make a paste of all the ingredients by just mixing them all together. Apply the paste on your face, making sure to avoid your eyes. Dip a small towel in warm water, and squeeze out the water. Place the towel on your face. Leave this for about 10 minutes. Using the towel gently clean of the mask, then pat dry.

Olive Oil- Pineapple Mask

Pineapple helps rid the skin of dead cells and dirt and also an excellent source of vitamin C. When used together with Olive oil, which is great for nourishing the skin and eliminating wrinkles.

You will need:
- 1 cup of Pineapple pieces
- 4 tsp of Olive oil

Directions:
Mash the pineapple and olive oil together either with fork or blender. Apply the mask on your face, neck, and other wrinkled body parts. Leave for 20 minutes and wash off with lukewarm water.

Curd and Turmeric Face Mask For Wrinkles

This homemade beauty tip for wrinkles will help to avoid any blemishes on the skin and also will protect your skin from wrinkles.

You need:
- Turmeric
- Curd

Direction:
Start by mixing a tablespoonful of curd and with a bit of turmeric. Gently apply the mixture on your face, and let it dry for 10 minutes. Rinse it off with lukewarm water.

Coconut Oil

Coconut oil is something that never lacks in my house, and it's undoubtedly the best moisturizer there is. Massaging a little drop on your face make all the difference. I recommend you rub it on your face before going to bed and wash off with warm water in the morning. The oil can also be used while bathing. Wet skin absorbs any moisturizer very well. Just before you pat dry your body after taking a bath, take a little coconut oil and apply all over your body. Now wash your body with water without using soap. Pat dry with a towel.

Turmeric- Sugarcane Mask

Turmeric is an age long beauty remedy for wrinkles. TURMERIC- SUGARCANE MASK has been used across Asia for centuries. In South Asia, they were an integral part of the bride's wedding preparations to making her look spotless and glamorous on her big day. They are known in Chinese and India traditions and are an element of the Ayurvedic medical system.

You will need:
- 2 tsp of Sugarcane juice- 2 tablespoons
- 2 tsp Turmeric

Directions:
- Mix sugarcane juice and turmeric thoroughly and apply on your face. Leave it for about 15 minutes before washing off with lukewarm water

Vitamin E Mask

Vitamin E contains antioxidant that helps fight free radicals thus inhibiting aging process and the formation of wrinkles. Vitamin E has a restorative property that helps repair and restore damaged cells. It moisturizing properties help prevent dull skin, and its natural cleaning feature helps clean dirt, debris and dead cells allowing the skin stay healthy.

You will need:
- 3 Capsules of Vitamin E capsules
- 2 tsp Yogurt
- ½ tsp Honey
- ½ tsp Lemon juice

Directions:
Extract the oil from vitamin E in a small bowl and add all other ingredients. Mix thoroughly and leave for about 10-15 minutes. Wash off with luke warm water.

Papaya, Banana, & Honey

Papaya is regarded as one of the best anti-wrinkle skin remedies. It is filled with vitamin C and E, and used primarily for growing wrinkles free skin. Banana acts as an excellent skin moisturizer to prevent dry skin.

Directions:
- Mash a slice of ripe papaya and half ripe banana with 2 tsp honey.
- Apply the mask on face and neck.
- Allow the mask to stand on skin for at least 20 minutes.
- Now wet your fingers with water and gently massage skin for 10 minutes befor washing off with lukewarm water.
- Repeat the process every day to prevent early signs of wrinkles and for a radiant completion.

• Homemade Ayurveda Anti-Wrinkle Moisturizer

I learned about this remedy from an old Ayurveda book. Although this treatment takes extra effort to put together, it's worth all the time and effort. Most people I recommended to use this recipe all gave positive feedbacks. This cream works well for wrinkles due to the presence of different oils for different skin types

You will need:

- 2 tsp Aloe vera gel
- Cocoa butter or lanolin- 1 oz. (approx. 30 ml or 2 tablespoons)
- Rosewater- 2 oz. (approx. 60 ml or 4 tablespoons)
  few drops of Lavender or rose essential oil
- One of the following oils as per your skin type- 3 oz.
  (approx. 90 ml or 6 table   spoons)
- Almond oil for healthy skin
- Sesame oil for dry skin
- Jojoba oil for oily and acne prone skin
- Rice bran oil or ghee (clarified butter) for mature skin
  (it is thin aging skin with dullness, uneven tone, fine lines and dry complexion)

Directions:

Heat up all the ingredients separately to make them warm. Then proceed to mix the warm ingredients with your blender. Whip the mixture well. While blending add the selected essential oil. Store the cream in a container and put in cool, dry place. Use this homemade moisturizer whenever you wash your face and at night when you go to sleep.

Below are few Facial Care Regime you need to know

- To add color to sallow skin, mash ½ cup of strawberry in a blender and apply them to your face. Leave them on for ten minutes, then rinse with tepid water.
- To alleviate puffiness in the eyes area, place cool cucumber slices over your eyes for ten minutes or more as needed
- To cleanse the pores, rub mashed tomato over your face
- To moisturize your skin, mash together grapes (a natural source of collagen and alpha-hydroxy acids) with enough honey to make a paste and apply the mixture to your face as a mask. Leave it in place for about twenty to thirty minutes while you relax, then rinse off
- To remove dead surface skin cells and improve skin texture, gently rub a small handful of dry short-grain rice against your face for a few minutes. Japanese women have used this technique for centuries

- To soften and nourish the skin, mash half of an avocado and apply it to your face. Leave it on until it dries, then rinse off with warm water. Avocado contains essential fatty acids and other nutrients that help prevent wrinkling
- To tighten and refine pores, whip up the white of an egg with a pinch of alum and apply it to your face as mask- After fifteen to twenty to twenty minutes, rinse it off with lukewarm water.

CHAPTER 29

Papaya for youthful skin

Mrs. Susan (My friend's mum) Introduced me to the power of papaya for the skin. Mrs. Susan is 50 years old and still rocking her ageless skin. Papaya is an excellent source of beta-carotene, filled with powerful enzymes and phytochemicals that are good for your skin. It's a good source of alpha-hydroxy acids, which exfoliates the skin and get rid of dark, dead skin cells. Papaya is rich in the enzyme papain. Papain is an enzyme that helps in skin lightening and reducing blemishes and acne scars. When consumed enriches the body with antioxidant, vitamin A, C and E which make your skin tight.

Nutrient	Benefit for Skin
Vitamin A	Helps heal and reduce acne visibility, scars, dark spots dry, flaky skin. Also, smoothens out aging skin.
Vitamin C	Helps boosts the production of collagen and promotes the elasticity and firmness.
Papain	Helps in skin lightening, decreases pigmentation, tones the skin and promotes skin regeneration. It also contains anti-inflammatory properties that help heal skin conditions like acne, rosacea, and eczema. Acts as a skin softener that smoothens out rough skin.
Alpha hydroxy acids	Help exfoliate the skin by breaking down bonds between dead cells
Potassium	Hydrates and moisturizes dry skin.

Note:

If you have sensitive skin, limit how you use papaya on your skin. The presence of the enzymes and alpha hydroxy acid might irritate your skin. In other to be on a safe side do a patch test on your inner elbow to confirm if the ingredient is safe for your skin.

Papaya for Acne

There are several ways to get rid of Acne with papaya. Firstly you can grind the green peel of papaya to form a consistent paste and apply the paste on your skin. You can as well mix the mask with a diluted vinegar solution and use on your skin. An alternatively is to make a more robust mask with honey, papaya, and lemon. This ingredient contains antibacterial properties which kill the acne causing bacteria. The honey available in the mask helps hydrate, exfoliate and soften your skin while preserving its moisture. Honey has antibacterial properties which starve acne causing bacteria and evens out any form of discolorations. The lemon acts as a natural astringent, which helps tighten pores and kill germs on the skin surface.

You need:
- ¼ ripe papaya
- 1 tablespoon honey
- 1/2 teaspoon lemon juice

Directions:

Using a blender blend soft papaya into a smooth, consistent paste. Add honey and lemon juice into the puree. Wash your fingers properly and use them to apply the paste on a clean face. Let it sit on your face for about 20 minutes. Then, gently loosen the mask with warm water before washing it off with cold. Pat your face dry and apply your favorite moisturizer. To make this mask more efficient, do a facial steaming before using the mask. Doing this will allow the mask penetrate deeply into your skin cells. Always go for raw organic honey if you want to get best results. Also, make sure that the lemon in use is fresh squeezed organic lemon not pasteurized.

Papaya, Cucumber Banana Facial Mask

I love to try out new things and see what works best. I have been using the cucumber and banana facial mask separately but this time, I decided to go wild and combine it with papaya and the result was fantastic. Cucumber helps hydrate, moisturize and cleanses the skin. Its skin lightening property helps clear blemishes and acne scars. When used as a mask helps relieves inflamed acne and sunburn. Banana, on the other hand, helps reduce wrinkles. It also promotes a glowing and vibrant skin – and play a huge role in hydrating your skin.

You need:
- ¼ ripe papaya
- ¼ cucumber
- ½ banana
- Blender

Directions:
You must have a blender before starting this mask. Firstly, peel all the ingredients and blend them all together to get a consistent puree. Do a facial steaming; this will allow your face absorb the mask better. Wash your hands properly and gently apply the mask on your face. Let the mask sit for about 20 minutes. It's now time to loosen the mask with warm water, then follow up by washing off with cold water. Pat dry and apply your favorite moisturizer. For best result use ripe papaya and banana.

Papaya and Egg White Face Mask

Several beauty recipes call for egg white. It tightens skin pores and removes excess sebum from the skin surface. It also does an excellent job in preventing acne and pimple.

You need:
- ¼ ripe papaya
- 1 egg white
- Blender

Directions:
Blend the papaya thoroughly to form a puree. Using a small bowl, whisk egg white in it, until it becomes frothy. Add the papaya puree into egg white and mix thoroughly. Wash your hands and apply the mask on your face. Let it sit for 15 minutes. Loosen the mask with warm water followed by cold water to close the pores.

Papaya and Milk cream

Milk contains lactic acid which helps lighten the skin and remedy sunburn or pigments. It also serves as an effective facial cleanser for the face, which will help keep your face fresh and glowing throughout the day. Raw milk contains beta hydroxy acid which is a natural exfoliant that removes dead skin. Milk is also effective in shrinking pores.

You need:
- ½ Raw Milk
- ¼ ripe papaya

Directions:

Start by blending your papaya in a blender, then add 1-2 tsp of milk and mix to form a smooth paste. Wash your hands and do your facial steam. Apply the paste on your face and neck. Let it sit for about 15-20 minutes, then wash off warm water, followed by cold water to close the pore. Pat dry

Wrinkles:

Papaya can also be used to diminish the appearance of wrinkles and crow's feet, due to the presence of its strong antioxidant. It's also rich in vitamin C, which helps ward off free radicals that damage the skin collagen and elastin.

You need
- ¼ papaya
- Olive oil

Directions:

You can do this by gently applying raw papaya puree around your eye. Let it sit for about 10 minutes before washing off. Do this daily to get rid of crow's feet. Alternatively, mix 1 tablespoon of ripe papaya puree with few drops of olive oil. Apply this mixture on affected area and let it sit for about 20 minutes. Wash off with cold water and use your choice of moisturizer.

Lightens Unwanted Facial Hair

Most people find facial hair very unattractive, if you are like this, worry no more – the papain enzyme present in raw papaya helps weaken the hair follicles on your face to prevent regrowth.

You need:
- ½ teaspoon of Turmeric powder
- ½ cups of raw papaya paste

Directions:

Start by making a puree of fresh papaya. Add ½ tablespoon of turmeric powder into the puree. Wash your fingers properly and apply the paste on the affected areas. Let it sit for about 20 minutes, by then it must have dried. Scrub off the paste and rinse your face with warm water followed by cold water to close your pores. Do this one every week for best results.

Heals Cracked Heels

In as much as your foot stays inside your shoes but most times. Many of us just don't want to see cracked heels. It sometimes causes flaky patches, itchiness, skin peeling, and bleeding. It might interest you to know that papaya is an excellent moisturizer and can help remedy cracked and dry heels.

You need:
- ¼ Papaya
- Olive oil

Directions:
Make a puree of papaya by blending it in a blender. Gently apply it on your cleaned heels. Let it sit for about 15 minutes. Now wash off and use olive oil. Repeat this daily before going to bed. Very soon you will start to see your feet becoming soft and smooth.

Controls Dandruff

Papaya contains enzymes that help prevent the build-up of oil and impurities on your scalp. It also plays a huge role in the treatment of dandruff. Yogurt's antibacterial properties fight the dandruff

You need:
- ½ cups of yogurt
- ¼ raw papaya

Directions:
Make a puree of papaya and add ½ cup of yogurt. Mix thoroughly and apply this mixture on your scalp. Let it sit for about 30 to 40 minutes before washing off with cold water. Finally, shampoo your hair. This remedy should be used once or twice daily for best results.

Alternatively, papaya can be used as a hair mask to nourish the hair. To make papaya mask, simply blend one cup of ripe papaya and ripe banana alongside with yogurt and 1 tablespoon of coconut oil. Apply this to your hair and cover up with a shower cap. Leave it on for 30 minutes before rinsing off. Use this mask once a week for a rapid result.

CHAPTER 30

Apple cider vinegar for Eczema

Some time in the past, I visited an old family friend, and it happened that his sister was down with eczema. My friend couldn't contain his excitement to see me. He said my coming to visit was a stroke of luck – his sister has been down with eczema for weeks; and plans are being made to take her to the hospital.

He had so much confidence that I have the solution to her eczema infection. Fortunately for me, I do. Firstly I need to say that I'm no miracle healer, I'm just a guy passionate about home remedies, so it drives me to read more about them. Eczema is not contagious; it's caused by a hypersensitivity reaction to an allergen. I have seen apple cider vinegar work in several cases of Eczema infections. I had no doubt about its efficacy. Fortunately for my friend there was a bottle of Apple Cider Vinegar lying around in the kitchen.

Why is vinegar so potent in the treatment of eczema?

- Vinegar is an excellent source of acetic, lactic and malic acids – which contains antibacterial and anti-fungal properties; that help fights skin infections, dry skin and relieves inflammation, itchiness, and dryness. Vinegar contains beta-carotene, which supports cell renewals.

- Vinegar is also an excellent source of potassium, which helps balance the pH level of your skin and deal with allergic situations.

- Vinegar is rich in a wide array of essential vitamins, minerals – which includes pectin, sodium, magnesium, potassium, iron, calcium, phosphorous, Sulphur and iron – all of which helps strengthen the immunes system and control eczema.

- It might also interest you to know that Apple cider vinegar is a rich source of fiber which is highly useful in flushing away of toxins that lead to eczema

Please dear ones, always use raw, organic, unfiltered and unpasteurized ACV – which usually appear dark and cloudy with sediments at the bottom of the bottle. So far the best brand I know of is the Bragg Organic Apple Cider Vinegar 32 oz

How to use Apple Cider Vinegar for Eczema

Apple cider vinegar can stand on its own or used in combination with another ingredient to remedy eczema. Below are various fun and easy ways to use Apple cider vinegar for eczema. You don't need to break the bank to do this. Just make do with some of the ingredients you can easily find in your kitchen

ACV Diluted in Water

If you can only lay your hands on ACV, there is nothing to worry about. It can do the work on its own, due to its antifungal and antibacterial properties. When applied to the eczema-affected skin, it gives instant relief.

You need:

- 2 Tsp Apple Cider Vinegar
- 1 Cup of Water
- 3 Cotton Balls

Directions:
Add a reasonable quantity of apple cider vinegar in a small bowl and add water to it. With the aid of a cotton swab apply the solution to the affected area. Repeat this remedy till you get the desired result. If you have a sensitive skin combine 1 tsp of apple cider vinegar with ½ water

Apple Cider Vinegar Bath

Having a vinegar bath has also proven to be very helpful with eczema. This remedy can also be taken a little bit further by adding sunflower oil to your bath water. Doing this helps treat the patches developed on the skin.

Your need:
- A bathtub
- ½ cups of Apple Cider Vinegar
- A Moisturizer

Directions:
Start by adding ACV to your bath water and gently soak yourself into it for about 15 minutes. Come out from the water and pat dry with a clean towel. After which you apply a moisturizer of your choice. Try your best to do this every day till you get your desired result

Taking ACV Orally

ACV can also be taken orally to help strengthen your immune system and prevent the reoccurrence of eczema. But remember always to dilute it before taking it orally. If you are suffering from heartburn or peptic ulcer, taking ACV orally is not advisable, because ACV is acidic and can cause you irritation.

You need:
- 1 tsp of Apple Cider Vinegar
- 1 Cup Water

Directions:
Dilute one tablespoon of Apple Cider Vinegar with 1 cup of water and drink this mixture afterward. This remedy should be followed at least 2 to 3 times daily to get rid of eczema and strengthen your immune system.

Apple Cider Vinegar and Baking Soda

I know you are eagerly expecting this combination. They both make for a potent combination and very useful in the treatment of eczema. The combination is ideal for creating a bacteria-unfriendly pH level.

You need:
- 2 tsp of Apple Cider Vinegar
- ¼ Baking Soda
- 1 cup Water

Directions:
Add 1 tsp of ACV to ¼ tsp of baking soda and mix with one cup of water. Stir the mixture thoroughly and drink this daily till you get rid of eczema. You can add 1 tsp of honey if you wish.

Apple Cider Vinegar and Honey

This combination is very effective in the cure of eczema – honey is well known for its ability to remedy skin diseases. When applied to the infected area can reduce inflammation and irritation. Its antibacterial properties also help kill harmful bacteria.

You need:
- 2 tsp of Apple Cider Vinegar
- 1 tsp Honey
- 1 glass of Water

Directions:
Add ACV and honey to one glass of water. Stir the mixture thoroughly and drink. This remedy should be taken three times daily with meals.

Additional tips:

- Dear ones, please for your safety please ensure you always dilute your ACV before taking it orally or topically. ACV is very strong and can cause severe burning sensation if taken without diluting it.

- It's best you avoid the usage of perfumes and other harsh soaps at the time being.

- If you are diabetic, I strongly advise you don't take ACV orally

- Before you use ACV. I suggest you do a simple test to ascertain if you are allergic to it. This can be done using a simple patch test. Apply a small amount to your skin and wait for a few minute

- If you are pregnant, please do not take ACV orally – because it can harm the little one

- Try as must as possible to keep your skin moisturize. Dry skin can significantly encourage eczema

- Food such as peanuts, milk, soy, wheat, fish and eggs should be avoided at the moment because it can worsen the situation.

- Please do take your health serious, your lifestyle does have a great impact on eczema. Eat more fresh fruits and vegetables. Try as possible to live a stress-free life.

- Take measure to stop constant sweating – frequent sweating can irritate your skin.

CHAPTER 31

Techniques to Prevent Premature Ejaculation

Premature ejaculation is defined as ejaculating in 4 minutes or less – or earlier than your partner wants or need for orgasm. The problem is becoming rampant with most men; as they run helter-skelter seeking for a quick fixes to this problem.

This issue has robbed most men of their ego and pride. I have received countless messages asking for the solution for PE. The truth is that nobody was born knowing how to last longer in bed. It is an art that should be learned and mastered. You shouldn't feel bad if you are not a professional in bed yet. Every expert was once an amateur. It's a known fact that women need longer time to reach orgasm than men. Most of the time they fake orgasm because they don't wish to harm their man's ego. While some will ask you to use your fingers to finish up the job. Personally, I have been in that position too, and I know how it feels. I have found that what worked for me the most was some series of exercise I did to strengthen my sexual muscles.

Types of Premature Ejaculation

Lifelong PE:

This starts earlier in life due to some bad habits, and it's usually very hard to treat. I have a friend who was a chronic masturbator as a child. He masturbated to ejaculate early, in order not to get caught. This early ejaculation act from masturbation caused him psychological issue which led to a lifelong PE.

Acquired PE:

This type of PE happens later in life and are often caused by psychological and physical issues like stress, diabetes or high blood pressure

Techniques to Delay Ejaculation
Self-Stimulation:

This method is all about practice and self-mastering. As awkward as it sounds, I recommend using masturbation to master this technique. Here you masturbate at least three times in a week for about 30 minutes and each time you are close to ejaculation hold it back and do not ejaculate. Do this at least six times during each session. The more you get close to the point of no return without actually giving in, the more familiar that sensation will be and the less urgency it will have.

Scrotal Pull:

If you have ever noticed, whenever you nears orgasm, your scrotum rises closer to your body. You can delay ejaculation by gently pulling your testes down and away from your body. Your partner can also do this for you. Doing this will buy you some good time.

Think Nonsexual Thoughts:

When you notice that you are beginning to get overly excited, it's time to turn off your thoughts to something you dislike. For me, I think about a car accident, lol, I so hate that scene. But don't over dwell on that thought. let's say 10 seconds, so you don't lose your erection. Then refocus your attention on your partner.

External Prostate Spot:

Do you know that men do have a G-spot? Yes, they do, and it's located about one inch below the rectum towards the scrotum. This spot can be reached by dipping your fingers into the anus till you reach that spot. But this can be tedious and can be passed across as been gay. But I have found that the second best way to reach this spot is stimulating the space between the anus and the back of the scrotum. This simple practice stimulates the male g-spot (prostate), the gland that supplies the fluid for semen during ejaculation. Whenever you are about to reach the point of no return, press on this spot firmly to block the ejaculatory reflex. This style also takes some amount of practice to discover the amount of pressure needed to ward of ejaculation and it also highly pleasurable.

Pc (Pubococcygeous) Muscle Contraction:

It works by squeezing your pelvic floor muscles around the scrotum, penis and anus as you are about to get to the point of no return. To perfect this before sex, simply, stop your urine stream mid-way while urinating and release after the count of three. Another way to exercise you PC muscle is to hold it for one or two seconds each time, then release. Repeat this three times a day, three to four times per week. Breathe normally during this exercise and try to avoid holding your breath.

The Squeeze Technique:

This method is quite straightforward to master and does not require any prior practice. Before you are about to ejaculate, pull out and squeeze the penis between the shaft and the glands (the pea-like junction just below the head) for 30 seconds. Although this can slightly make you lose your erection, but it will certainly stop the ejaculation while you stimulate yourself back and get back into business.

Breathing:

Deep breathing helps control the arousal and tension that leads to early ejaculation. Inhale for 5 seconds, hold it for about three seconds and exhale for about five seconds, then start all over again. If you apply this breathing technique without breaking the rhythm during intercourse, it will drastically slow down your ejaculation. This technique helps relieve performance anxiety and lower your arousal to level that easy to control.

Focus on Foreplay:

Who says you can't satisfy your partner if you have PE? You can still make her cum by stimulating her genital organs. My ex-girlfriend will always make me thrust my thighs in-between her vulva while she moves swiftly. If you can go down on her, knock yourself out. Feel free to ask her what she wants.

Take It Slow:

You are rushing to nowhere; her pus*** isn't running away. Take it slowly. Slow and gentle movement can hold off orgasm. Whenever you find yourself getting close to orgasm, slow down a bit. Try changing your position. Or trying stimulating your partner with other ways.

CHAPTER 32

Effective Remedies for Kidney Stones

Kidney stones are caused by the accumulations of mineral salts, which lodge anywhere along the course of the urinary tract.

These stones can sometimes form in the bladder or kidney. Causing severe pain. Our urine is often saturated with uric acid, phosphates, and calcium oxalate but due to the secretion of various protective compounds and natural mechanisms that help control the pH of our urine, these substances remain suspended in solution. Sometimes when the protective compound is overwhelmed, these substances may crystallize and begin to clump together and eventually forming large stones enough to restrict urinary flow.

Some Symptoms Includes:

- Severe pain radiating from the upper back to the lower abdomen and groin
- Profuse sweating,
- Frequent urination
- Blood in the urine
- Odor or cloudy urine
- Absence of urine formation
- Nausea and vomiting

Kidney stone is more common in white men than black men. There are four kinds of kidney stone: Calcium stone, uric acid stone, struvite stone and cysteine stone. The majority of kidney stone are calcium stones. High blood calcium can lead to hypercalciuria, which is the excessive absorption of calcium from the intestine. Thereby increasing the level of calcium in the urine.

Kidney stone usually cause no symptoms until they are dislodged. A dislodged kidney stone can cause severe pain in the flank or kidney area.

Recommendations

- Reduce consumption of refined carbohydrates, foods rich in white sugar and flour
- Reduce alcohol consumption and increase fiber intake
- Lessen the intake of lots of saturated fats
- Lessen the consumption of animal protein foods.
- *Avoid foods high in oxalate content:* Oxalate when combined with calcium and iron form crystals that may be excreted in urine or form larger kidney stones that can block the kidney tubules. Examples of foods high in oxalate are peanuts, almonds, wheat bran, spinach, black tea, cashews, hazelnuts, soybeans, soy milk, instant tea, rhubarb, beets, sweet potatoes, most dried beans and chocolate.
- People with kidney stone are advised to lessen foods with much salt and sodium.
- I also strongly recommend you drink a lot of water. Inadequate fluid intake influences the accumulation of crystals in the urine. I suggest you take 8 to 10 glasses of water daily. It will also make your urine clear, which is a good sign.

Tip: Drinking a glass of water before bed, during the night when you're still awake and before going back to bed

Below are Some Home Remedies for Kidney Stones:

Watermelon:

Watermelon is one of the best vegetables for kidney stones, due to its high water content. Also, the high potassium content in watermelon is believed to help in dissolving kidney stones. Eating watermelon on a regular basis will help prevent and treat kidney stone. Below is a simple juice recipe for kidney stone:

Kidney Stone Juice
- 1 orange, peeled
- 1 apple
- 1 lemon
- 4 slices of watermelon
- 4 ice cubes

Aloe Vera:

Aloe Vera contains aloemannan, which slows the rate of crystal formation. Take ¼ cup daily (Please do not use for more than two weeks at a time) Aloe Vera prevents deposition of free radicals and helps impede the formation of kidney stones. Regular consumption or aloe Vera juice helps in reducing kidney stones.

Apple Cider Vinegar:

Apple Cider vinegar is very robust in dissolving kidney stones. And also has a great alkalinizing effect on the blood and urine
Mix two tablespoons of organic apple cider vinegar and one teaspoon of honey in one cup of warm water.
Drink this a few times a day.

Lemon Juice and Olive Oil:

The citric acid present in lemon helps break down calcium stones and hinder further growth. This particular remedy has recorded remarkable growth in the treatment of gallbladder stones, but can also be used to treat kidney stones.
- Add equal amount of fresh lemon juice and olive oil, mix and drink
- After which you take plenty water.
- Do this two to three times a day, up to three days. You need not continue this remedy if you can pass the stones in a single dose.

If you have a family history of kidneys stone, I suggest you take calcium supplements with meals. When calcium rich foods with oxalates are consumed, they bind together and are expelled in the stool, which lessens your risk of kidney stone. Remember this is only applicable for people with kidney stone history in their families.

Pomegranate

Pomegranate juice is high in antioxidant and helps protect you against health risks, such as kidney stones, blood cholesterol, and hypertension. They are rich in polyphenols, which are antioxidant that helps protect the body from free radicals which make it excellent for your kidney. The seeds and juice of pomegranates have astringent properties that can assist in the treatment of kidney stones. For optimum result drink freshly made pomegranate daily. Another great option is to grind one tablespoon of pomegranate seed into a fine paste. Consume the paste with a cup of horse gram, once daily. This remedy goes a long way to dissolve kidney stone

Try to eat one whole pomegranate or drink one glass of freshly squeezed pomegranate juice daily. You can mix pomegranate in a fruit salad also.

Another option is to grind one tablespoon of pomegranate seeds into a fine paste. Eat this paste along with a cup of horse gram soup once daily. This remedy will help dissolve the stones. You can find horse gram in Indian markets.

Nettle Tea

Nettle tea is well known to help remedy kidney stone because it acts as a kidney flushing agent. When treating kidney stone, some herbalists recommends two cups of infused nettle tea daily for ten to twelve weeks or longer.

For best effect try a cup of nettle tea daily for six weeks. After which you can make it three cups a week. Nettle tea should not be taken after 5 pm due to its diuretic effect, which can interfere with a good night sleep. The diuretic effect helps flush the kidneys and the digestive system.

Nettle Leaf

Nettle Leafs helps maintain the flow of water through the kidneys and bladder, thus, promote easy urination. Nettle leafs also prevent crystals from forming into stones and keeps bacteria away.

How to Make a Nettle Infusion

Nettle infusion is the most potent water-based herbal preparation. The infusion should be steeped overnight.

Procedure:
- Use organic stinging nettles
- Put one heaped tablespoon of dried nettle in a quart mason jar
- Pour hot water over the nettles leaves
- Close the jar and leave till day break
- Then strain out the leaves, the mixture should appear dark green in color
- Add 1/4 cup lemon juice (optional)
- Sweeten with honey (optional)
- Drink two to three cups of nettle tea daily for at least 3 weeks

Basil

Research has shown that taking basil tea can significantly enhance the general well-being of your kidney. Basil also helps induce stone expulsion from the urinary tract, and it's regarded as a kidney tonic.

Procedure:
- Use organic basil
- Pour hot water into a mason jar and soak the leaves
- Close the jar and leave it to stay overnight
- Strain out the leaves
- Mix with honey
- Take two teaspoon
- Soak leaves of basil in water and leave overnight. Extract juice from them and add honey to it and drink. One teaspoon of the juice is a right dosage. Eating basil leaf raw after washing them properly is also helpful.

Wheatgrass

Wheatgrass is highly potent in the treatment of kidney stones and other diseases naturally. Mix one teaspoon of lemon juice with wheatgrass juice and basil leaves. Wheatgrass juice is highly effective in treating kidney stones and other kidney diseases naturally. You can also have a glass of wheatgrass juice mixed with one teaspoon each of lemon juice and juice extracted from basil leaves.Take it two to three times a day. Wheatgrass juice is a good source of magnesium, potassium, iron, amino acids, chlorophyll, and B vitamins.

Celery

Celery is known for its diuretic properties which help flush out toxins and depositions from the kidney and urinary tract. A cup of celery juice helps clear toxins that contribute to the formation of kidney stones. Regular intake of celery juice prevents kidney stones from forming. The seeds are also used in the treatment of kidney stone. Drinking the herbal tea made with celery seeds can help treat kidney stone resulting from uric acid.

Tomatoes

Tomatoes are high in lycopene, which is a potent antioxidant known to prevent serum lipid oxidation and formations of kidney stones. To use this remedy, make a juice of tomatoes and add a little pepper and salt to it.

Kidney Beans

kidney bean is high in fiber and is useful in the treatment of kidney and bladder problems.
Procedure:
- Detach the beans from the pod
- Put the beans in hot water.
- Simmer the water in low flame for hours until the beans become soft and tender.
- Strain the liquid out
- Drink the liquid from the beans several times throughout the day to relieve kidney stone pain.

NB:
The liquid should not be kept for more than 24 hours so as the maintain its therapeutic value

Bran Flakes

High intake of fiber foods is recommended for people suffering from kidney stone. The fiber will help rid of the excess calcium in the urine, thereby cutting down the risk of kidney stones.
Procedure:
- Pour two cups of Bran Flakes into a bowl
- Eat in the morning, to reduce risk of kidney stone

Others:

In general, foods with high antioxidant properties are helpful in the treatment of kidney stones. Some of the food with highest antioxidant properties include artichoke, Grapes, black bean dried, black plum, blackberry, blueberry, dried red kidney bean, gala apple, granny smith apple, sweet cherry, pecan, pinto bean, plum, prune, raspberry, Onions, red apple, and Coconut water.

CHAPTER 33

Home Remedies for Removing Gallstones

One faithful Saturdays morning, one of my clients called me in a distressed tone. I could hardly hear what she was saying, so I opted to call her back when she is more relaxed. After a while, I called her back. With teary voice, she told me that lately she has been feeling a rapid intensifying pain on the top right portion of her abdomen and severe back pain between her shoulders. After explaining to her doctor, he ran regular checks on her and recommended surgery to remove her gallbladder.

May I inform you that when doctors take out the gallbladder, which is a major surgery, they usually take out the appendix too – in essence, you lose two vital organs. Although there is no risk associated with the surgery, the thought of going under the knife terrified her.

Let me cut the long story short. She didn't go for the surgery, but rather she followed my gallstones remedy to dissolve her gallstones. If you haven't had any encounter with this disease, you might be wondering, what the hell are gallstones? Gallstones are simply those hard deposits that form inside the gallbladder. The gallbladder is a small, pear-shaped organ on the right side of your abdomen, just beneath your liver. Gallstones can sometimes range from the size of a grain to as large as a golf ball – mostly formed by the development of too much cholesterol in the bile secreted by the liver. Below are a few other causes

- **Concentrated bile:** A situation where your gallbladder fails to empty the bile content, and the bile becomes overly concentrated and causes a stone.

- **Bilirubin:** Bilirubin is a chemical produced when the liver destroys old red blood cells. Stones form when your gallbladder cannot break down the excess bilirubin. Let's dive straight in the home remedies for gallstone.

Home Remedies for Removing Gallstones

Instead of going under the knife and getting your gallbladder removed – in which you lose two vital organs, the gallbladder, and the appendix; why don't you save yourself the pain and the money and do a simple effortless cleanse. The cleanse takes four days to complete. It's straightforward and inexpensive. The primary ingredient in this cleanse is the apple juice.

The Gallbladder Cleanse:

Get your juicer ready because this is going to be a bumpy ride. Visit the grocery store and purchase the below produce in advance before the cleanse.
- One big container, filled with apples, enough to make 4 gallons of apple juice
- 4 gallons of steam distilled water
- 1/2 virgin olive oil or cold-pressed peanut oil
- 3 lemons (or enough to make 1/4 cup lemon juice)

- Tomatoes for Tomato juice
- 1 straw (optional)

Upon waking up every morning, prepare one gallon of apple juice – which you will be drinking every day for the 4 days, coupled with a gallon of distilled water. Every morning or evening for the 4 days do a coffee enema – this will help expel the toxins which are being deposited in your rectum.

Drinking Oil

At night before you retire to bed, drink ½ cups of virgin olive oil or peanut oil, not refined. I will advise you first to chill the oil a little bit, so it gets cold (always sip with a straw to minimize its unpleasantness) Follow it up with ¼ cup of fresh squeezed lemon juice. Now its time to lie down, but sleep on your right side with two pillows under your right hip. The purpose is to slant the body so that the oil wouldn't leave the stomach faster and go into the duct area and to the gallbladder. While you rest, the oil will saturate and cleanse the body tissues.

Reactions to Cleanse

The usual reaction that is accompanied by drinking oil and lemon is burping or vomiting. But when this starts I suggest you sip a bit of tomato juice. Some nights you may vomit or be nauseated – this is usually caused by the gallbladder ejecting the stones with such force that it shoots the oil back into the stomach, when the oil returns to your stomach, you get sick. Be ready to experience a night of discomfort, after all, it's nothing compared to the recovery from surgery that involves many months of pain and suffering. You may experience a discharge of stones which usually comes like a sharp pain and mild contraction.

The Fourth Day (Passing the Stone)

During the fourth day you might begin to experience a bowl movement – go to the toilet and have a lovely time. Trust me, it wouldn't be as painful as you think, the oil will make them slick, and the lemon juice takes the sharpness away – making them soft when passed. Take out time to look inside the toilet; you might see the stones floating near the top of the toilet water. The stones usually come in different sizes; some are as tiny as a pebble while some can be as big as your thumb. They also come in various shades of green and may be bright colored and shiny like gemstones. The color comes from the bile. The light colored ones are the newest – the blackish stones are the oldest. That's the reason why most people will tell you they saw what seems to look like balls of bright green grass. After passing the gallstone, you will experience increased stamina. Don't back out now and get excited yet, there is still more cleansing work to be done. Don't be quick to get back to your regular food, start by introducing plenty fruits and vegetable into your diet and continue with the coffee enema. Below is the juice therapy I strongly recommend for you after the cleanse.

Beetroot, Cucumber and Carrot Juice for Gallstones

Beetroot, cucumber, and carrots are highly effective for gallbladder cleanse. Cucumber, with its high water content, is great for detoxifying the liver as well as the gallbladder. Beets strengthens and cleanses gallbladder and liver. It also helps in cleansing the colon and your blood. Carrot juice is high in vitamin C and other nutrients, which also detoxifies the gallbladder.

Get this:
• 1 Beet root
• 1 Cucumber
• 1 Carrots (medium)

Directions:
Start by washing your produce thoroughly. Then slice them into bits. Put them down your juicers chute. Enjoy you sweet red juice. You can add apples, celery, and ginger while making the juice. I suggest you put an extra detoxification effort and go on another a 2 days juice fast, using the recipe mentioned above.

Apple Juice and Apple Cider Vinegar for Gallstones

Like my grandmother will always say, an apple a day keeps you away from the doctor. Apple is an excellent source of malic acid which helps to soften the gallstones and makes it easy to remove. While apple cider vinegar help inhibit the liver in making cholesterol and reduce pains associated with the stone. Both are used together in dissolving gall stones. This is done by mixing apple cider vinegar with a glass of apple juice.

Get this:
• 1 Glass of Apple Juice
• 1 tablespoon of Apple Cider Vinegar

Directions:
Juice your apple with a juicer and mix the apple juice with apple cider vinegar. Mix thoroughly and drink every day. I also recommend that you eat your apple

regularly. Another great way to use apple cider vinegar is to combine 2 tablespoons of ACV with 1 tsp of lemon juice – diluted with a glass of water. This mixture should be drank on empty stomach first thing in the morning upon waking up

Pear Juice

There are broad claims on the web that pear juice can help remedy gallstone. These claims are virtually everywhere that you can't afford to overlook them. Most people swore to it. I haven't tried it or recommended it yet, but pear juice would never harm you. The idea behind it is that pectin contained in the pear juice binds to cholesterol-filled gallstones and helps move them out of your body. Most herbalist I know, recommends pear juice for liver or gallbladder flush along with other oil and herb. Below is a simple home remedy that calls for pear juice and honey you can use.

Ingredients:
- ½ glass Pear juice
- ½ glass Hot water
- 2 tsp Honey

Directions:
Add the pear juice and honey into a glass of hot water. Stir thoroughly until the honey dissolves completely. Drink this thrice daily to prevent gallstones.

Milk Thistle for Gallstones

Yes, milk thistle works, I know because I prescribed it to a client and she gave me positive feedback. A clinical trial performed at New York University Langone Medical Center proves that a component found in milk thistle, known as silymarin helps protect against gallbladder stone formation. There are several ways to include milk thistle into your diet. I usually recommend that my clients add the powdered milk thistle seed to their juices, salads, vegetables or make tea with it.
Below is a simple recipe.

Get this
- 1 tsp Milk thistle leaves and seeds (you may even use packaged tea)
- 1 Muslin bag (Get yours here)
- 1 cup Hot water
- Honey (optional)

Directions:
Start by crushing milk thistle leaves and seeds in the muslin bag. Place the bag in hot water and steep for about 5 minutes – add honey and mix thoroughly, then sipDAN

Dandelion for Gallstones

Dandelion sure do work in eliminating gallstones; this is because it helps encourage the excretion of bile from the liver, so the body can properly metabolize fat. Another way it contributes to the dissolution of gallstones is by revitalizing sluggish gallbladder which duty is to store and excrete bile as needed by the body. So, it does make perfect sense to use dandelion to cure gallstones. The tender leave can also be added to salads or steamed. It is also available in capsule form.

Get this:
- 1 cup Hot water
- 1 tsp Dried dandelion leaves
- Honey (optional)

Directions:
Put the dandelion leaves in a bowl and pour hot water into it. Cover and leave it to steep for 5 minutes. Add honey if you wish. Drink this tea twice or thrice daily. If you suffer from diabetes, consult your doctor before taking the dandelion herb.

Lemon Juice for Gallstone

If you read the beginning of this, chapter, I talked about the four days cleanse. Lemon is one of the vital ingredients. Lemon helps stop your liver from making cholesterol. Simply, add the juice of half a lemon in a glass of water and have it twice or thrice a day. Alternatively, you can try the below Ayurveda remedy using lemon juice to dissolve your gallstones.

Get this:
- 30 ml Olive oil
- 30 ml Fresh lemon juice-
- 5g Garlic paste

Directions:
Make a mixture of olive oil, lemon juice, and garlic paste. Drink this mixture every day upon waking up – on an empty stomach, for at least 40 days.

Psyllium:

A naturopathic doctor friend of mine will always suggest you increase your intake of fiber, which primary source are fruits and vegetables. One of his most recommended herbs is Psyllium – which is a form of fiber made from the Plantago ovata plant, specifically from the husk of the plant's seed, and mostly known as a laxative. Psyllium acts as an excellent remedy for gallstones and helps bind the cholesterol in the bile and thus preventing the formation of gallstones. When taken regularly will help to avoid constipation and other causes of gallstone formation.

Ingredients:
- 1 tsp Psyllium powder husk
- 1 glass of Water

Directions:
Add psyllium to water, stir thoroughly and drink the solution. I suggest you drink this at night before going to bed every night. Make sure to drink plenty of water after taking it – because it absorbs water a lot and can make you feel dehydrated.

Peppermint for Gallstones

Peppermint oil is choleretic, which simply implies that it encourages bile secretion from the liver. It is used in a formula with other terpenes to help dissolve gallstones. Because peppermint oil is rapidly absorbed into the bloodstream from the stomach, studies have concluded that enteric-coated capsules of peppermint oil deliver the benefit directly to the intestines, rather than to the stomach. Peppermint tea is very useful when you have that gallbladder attack. It helps relax spasms and relieve you from acute pain.

Get this:
- 1 tsp Fresh or dried mint leaves
- 1 tsp Water
- Honey (optional)

Directions:
Start by crushing the mint leaves, keep them aside. Boil water and add the crushed mint leaves inside. Put off the flame and cover it. Let it steep for about 3-5 minutes. Strain and add honey. Have this tea in between meals.

Diet Tips for Gallstones

- Increase your intake of fruits and vegetables. Fresh fruit and vegetable contain fiber which helps encourage bowel evacuation of small gallstones

- Go on a regular juice fast – dong this supports liver detoxification while cleansing the system and providing Vitamin C. Feel free to do your coffee enema while on the fast. I suggest you include beetroot, carrot, celery and ginger in your fast

- Eat lots of fresh fruits, especially apples. Apples have an affinity for binding to excess cholesterol.

- Begin your day with a glass of warm water with ½ lemon squeezed in it. Lemon juice stimulates digestive and liver function, cleanse the bowels and has a beneficial effect.

- Lecithin sprinkled on your food, cereal or in a smoothie helps to emulsify fats, lipids and oils and the breakdown of cholesterol and bile in the digestion due to the phosphatidylcholine

- Maintain a diet low in cholesterol. Doing this will greatly help prevent gallstones. A low cholesterol diet takes the strain off your liver and gall bladder.

- Bitter food stimulates liver and gallbladder function. I suggest you increase your intakes of food like kale, endive, radicchio and endive. Food high in Sulphur should also be encouraged. These foods help stimulate liver detoxification, they include garlic, Brussels Sprout, Cabbage, Onion, Broccoli, Cauliflower, and Radish.

- Go for the good raw oil. These oils can be derived from food like raw olive oil, fish oil capsules, flaxseed oil capsules, fish, nut, and seeds.

- Intake of Omega 3 essential fatty acids should be increased. You can easily get this from Mackerel, Anchovies, Cod, Sardine, Snapper, Sardines and Halibut.

- Reduce intake of saturated fats (animal fats and dairy foods), Trans-fatty acids, processed foods and simple sugars. Saturated fats and Trans-fatty acids are commonly found in foods such as cakes, cookies, biscuits, bakery foods, margarine, donuts, processed and deep fried foods.

- Herbs such as Dandelion, Burdock, Peppermint, Green Tea, Lemon, and Ginger should be taken. These herbs support detoxification, digestion and bile production.

CHAPTER 34

Alternative Treatment for Yeast Infection

A friend of mine recently approached me for a remedy to cure vaginal yeast infection. The fact that she confided in me with something as personal as that, made me willing to go the extra mile to compile this lengthy piece on vaginal yeast infection.

This piece will also serve as a guide for all those suffering from yeast infection. To fully understand vaginal yeast infection, it imperative you know that yeast is a microorganism which is found in the body in smaller quantity. The Lactobacillus bacteria produces acid that help prevents the overgrowth of yeast. It becomes a problem when there is a balance disruption, and too many yeast cells start growing in the vagina – which may lead to itching, burning accompanied with soreness and redness. In some cases, the woman might experience white clumpy vaginal discharge along with pain during intercourse and urination. This condition is what is known as yeast infection and it's medical name is well known as Candidiasis. This overgrowth can most times result from pregnancy, uncontrolled diabetes, the use of oral contraceptives, which increases the estrogen level and the use of antibiotic which can decrease lactobacillus bacteria in the vagina.

Although, yeast infection is considered a sexually transmitted disease. Women who aren't sexually active can still contact the disease. Women are not only alone in this. Men also suffer from penile yeast infection but not at the rate women do. But most likely among men who aren't circumcised. The symptoms in men are red rashes on their penis along with itching or burning sensation on the tip of the penis. The good news is that yeast infection can be cured either by medication or home remedies. I will always advise you go for home remedies.

Powerful Home Remedies for Vaginal Yeast Infection

Yogurt Remedy for Yeast

Yogurt contains Lactobacillus acidophilus, a bacterium that's found in healthy vaginas and known to help kill the yeast infection by producing hydrogen peroxide. Yogurt is also known to help restore the balance between good and bad bacteria while reducing the irritation. The presence of good bacteria in yogurt interacts with the sugar found in your diet while attacking the yeast. This process generates hydrogen peroxide through the chemical process of fermentation. Yogurt is an excellent source of probiotic which helps cure the yeast infection and also helps maintain the balance of good bacteria.

Directions:
- Endeavor to eat plain yogurt daily.
- You can also apply yogurt liberally in and around your vagina. A simple way to do this is to soak a cotton ball in yogurt. With the soaked cotton wool apply the yogurt all over the affected areas. Leave for about 20 – 30 minutes before washing off with water. Then pat dry. Buttermilk also has the same effect as yogurt and can be drunk twice daily in place of yogurt.

Garlic Treatment

Garlic works pretty well in the treatment of yeast infection. I have seen it work in tons of different occasions. Try this simple experiment, while baking bread add garlic while the dough is rising, it will kill the yeast instantly. The trick with using garlic to remedy yeast infection is to catch the infection earlier – the first day you notice a slight, fleeting tickle or itchiness. Which is usually followed by the white and lumpy like tiny bit of cottage cheese. When this happens, take a clove of fresh garlic and peel off the natural paper shell that covers it – while leaving the clove intact, insert it into the vagina and leave overnight. One night treatment can be enough to kill the infection. If symptoms persist, continue for one or two more days till the itchiness are all gone. This treatment is best done at bedtime, because there is a connection between the mouth and the vagina, and when placed inside the vagina the taste travels up the mouth. Do note that upon waking up the odor emanating from your mouth will be unpleasant. In some severe cases where the woman has large quantities of white discharge and red sore labia; cut the garlic in half before inserting it into the vagina. Any cut in the clove will make the treatment stronger.

Grapefruit Seed Extract for Yeast Infection

I have seen this make rounds on the web, and most people swore that grapefruit seed extract worked for them. According to diagnoseme.com a website overseen by medical doctors – states that the natural antibiotic found in grape fruit can kill a wide variety of pathogens along with bacteria and protozoa. Grapefruit seed extract is known to have a natural antibiotic, and anti-fungal properties that help kills the growing yeast.

Directions:
- Start by adding 5 – 10 drops of grapefruit seed extract to 2 cups of water.
- Dissolve it thoroughly inside the glass of water.
- Soak a cotton ball in the water and apply it on the infected area.
- Do this daily consistently for three days.
- **A word of caution:** If you are pregnant or menstruating I strongly advise against this remedy. Also, if you notice any form of irritation discontinue usage.

Coconut Oil for Yeast Infection

The chapter on coconut oil took me over three months to write because I wanted to gather as much information I can about the miraculous oil. When it comes to coconut oil – yeast infection doesn't stand a chance. Most research conducted on this subject sure proves that the medium chain fatty acid found in coconut oil is effective in killing Candida yeast. Coconut oil contains 3 different fatty acids (Caprylic Acid, Capric Acid, Lauric Acid) that have each been found to be effective against the Candida yeast. The caprylic acid being the most potent ingredient against candida kills the yeast cells by interfering with their cell walls. Both capric acid and lauric acid have powerful antifungal treatments – making it impossible for candida yeast to build up resistance against coconut oil – unlike other antifungals which lose their effectiveness over time. Caprylic Acid being one of the three fatty acids found in coconut oil is very potent in killing candida cells and restoring stomach acidity to its normal state. According to a study conducted by Japan's Niigata University, "the fungicidal effect of caprylic acid on Candida Albicans was exceedingly powerful.

How to Use Coconut Oil for Yeast Infection (Topical Application)

Get this:
- Coconut oil
- Cotton ball

Directions:
Take a cotton ball and soak it in coconut oil and gently wipe the infected areas with the soak cotton ball. Repeat this thrice daily for best results. If you feel any sticky sensation wipe the oil dry with a soft cloth after about 30 minutes

2nd Method

Get this:
- Virgin coconut oil, preferably organic- 3-5 tbsp

Directions:
Simply take a tablespoon of coconut oil with every meal – breakfast, lunch and dinner. Which equates to 3 tablespoons daily – enough to counter yeast infection. If the yeast infection is severe – feel free to take more. Coconut is natural and harmless to the body, which means you can take it as much as you like. You can also add it to your toast, salads, and smoothies.

3rd Method

Get this:
- 3-4 tbsp Coconut oil
- 8 cups Warm water

Directions:
- Start by adding coconut oil into a warm bowl of water. Stir thoroughly and use it to rinse your vagina

Essential Oils for Yeast Infection

There are several essential oil with strong anti-bacterial, anti-viral and anti-fungal properties which can also be used to remedy yeast infection. These oils are tea tree oil, cinnamon oil, and grape seed oil, all of which are very powerful in fighting candida infections. Below is a simple recipe to make a potent concoction using some essential oils with carrier oils – to give you instant relief from the infection.

Get this:
- 2 tbsp Grapeseed oil – carrier oil
- 2-3 drops Tea tree oil.
- 2-3 drops Cinnamon oil.
- 2-3 drops Oregano oil.
- 2-3 drops Peppermint oil.
- 2-3 drops Lemon oil.

Directions:
Mix all the oils together and store in a bottle. Using a soaked cotton ball apply the oil on the affected area. Let it sit for a few minutes. Wipe off with clean soft cloth. Repeat this process twice daily.

Vinegar for Yeast Infection

Apple Cider Vinegar helps restore the vagina pH level and prevents yeast fungi from thriving and infecting the vagina with further yeast infections. It is one of nature's strongest antibiotics that kills bacteria, viruses, and protozoa providing instant relief. ACV helps to re-colonize the intestines and vagina with friendly bacteria which acts as a dominant guard to stop the harmful bacteria (Candida) from returning.

Directions: (ACV in Diet)
- Try as much as possible to include apple cider vinegar in your diet, this helps prevent yeast infection by maintaining proper pH balance hindering fungal growth.
- Regular intake also boosts the immune system, fight against Candida – helps good bacteria and prevents yeast infection.

Method 1
- 1 tsp of ACV can be mixed with a glass of water or herbal tea. Drink this regularly 2 – 3 times daily on an empty stomach to prevent yeast infection.
- Take ACV in supplement form as tablets, capsules, or in tonic form.

Method 2

- Start by soaking a clean cloth or cotton balls in diluted ACV for 2 – 3 minutes – place the cloth on the walls of the vagina. Repeat this regularly until yeast infection is gone

CHAPTER 35

Untold Psoriasis Treatment, Revealed!

Psoriasis is a chronic inflammatory disease of the skin in which the skin cells proliferate and shed at an abnormal rate. Its causes do not originate from the surface but within the intestinal tract. Psoriasis is an ugly disease and can significantly dampen your self-esteem.

Recently I read about a severe case where a young girl by the name Giorgia Lanuzza, who was diagnosed with psoriasis at the age of 13 after her father died. I have also witnessed several cases while working alongside with my grandmother in her healing center.

These events and the inquiries I get most of the times motivated me to do a thorough research on the disease.

Firstly, if you are down with psoriasis, water should be your best friend. Water helps in ridding your body of toxins, so they don't keep pouring out through your skin.

Dr. Pagano strongly recommends you drink six to eight ounces of water and eat a serving or two a day of stewed figs, apples, raisins, apricots, pear, peaches, or prunes because their laxative effect helps clean your bowels.

Many physicians will tell you that psoriasis has no cure, but that's a fat lie. I have followed Dr. Pagano for years now and have carefully observed his processes. In his words "When you understand the real cause of psoriasis, you will know that the disease can is curable with a natural approach" For more on his process I suggest you buy his bestselling book called Healing Psoriasis: The Natural Alternative

According to Dr. Pagano's research, the treatment lies in avoiding certain foods that contributed to "leaky gut" and taking two natural teas on a daily basis.

Slippery ELM

In his book, he states that the herb slippery elm helps coat the inner lining of the intestinal wall while promoting healing.

Directions:
- Pour a ½ teaspoon of slippery elm powder in a cup of warm water, leave it for 15 minutes and stir. Drink afterward.
- Don't eat for the next 10 minutes. Repeat this every day for the next ten days of the program and every other day. Psoriasis should gradually clear.

American Yellow Saffron Herbal Tea.

In his book, he states that the American yellow saffron tea helps heal the lining of the intestinal walls as it flushes the liver and kidney of toxins.

Directions
Pour a ¼ teaspoon of saffron in a cup, then add boiling water and leave it for about 15 minutes. Drink this five days a week till psoriasis clears

Psoriatrax

If you ask me to recommend the best shampoo for psoriasis, it will be PsoriaTrax. I will like to call this a fail proof shampoo for psoriasis. My buddy Israel tried it on his psoriasis scalp and the result was just fantastic. He couldn't believe his eyes and immediately rushed down to my house to testify to the product. I was quiet impressed myself, so I decided to do a background search on it. I searched for the product on amazon and discovered it has well enough positive reviews from people who have used it.

The active ingredient in PsoriaTrax is coal tar. Coal tar is approved by the FDA for the treatment of psoriasis. Coal tar is a derivative of coal and wood (juniper, pine) and has well used for medicinal purposes for hundreds of years. The properties in coal tar go to work in two ways:
Coal tar is thought to naturally inhibit DNA replication of skin cells; slowing down the buildup of excess skin cells, thereby significantly reducing the scaling and thickening of skin.
Coal tar breaks down keratin, the protein which is the "building block" for skin structure. This helps the excess skin cells (the dry, scaly patches) on the skin surface to break up and shed more easily.
As an added benefit, coal tar offers some anti-itch and anti-inflammatory effects. Generally, the higher the concentration of tar, the more effective the product.

Directions
- For Psoriasis patches on the skin, apply either formula of PsoriaTrax shampoo to affected areas and rinse off. Use PsoriaTrax Coal Tar Glide throughout the day. It comes in a very portable stick with a unique Glide Head applicator for complete coverage for large and small areas. PsoriaTrax Glide can be applied alone or over a moisturizer.
- Coal tar makes skin more sensitive to sunlight, so be sure to use a sunscreen. Tar remains active on the skin for at least 24 hours, and you are at increased risk of sunburn during this period.

Fish Oil

The omega-3 content of fish oil or flaxseed oil helps heal the compromised intestinal walls and their possible role in inflammation.

Tunn off the Nightshade:

Patients living with psoriasis should avoid plants in the nightshade family. It is mandatory that you stay away from these plants if you want to heal. These plants includes:

- Tomatoes
- Peppers (all Capsicum species including bell, hot and pimento peppers and all foods made from these peppers including paprika, cayenne pepper, and Tabasco sauce)
- Eggplant

- Ground cherries
- Tomatillos
- Garden huckleberries
- Tamarillos
- Pepinos
- Naranjillas.

Tomato is the worst of all and should be avoided as much as possible and that includes other tomatoes based food like ketchup and tomato juice. Anything with tomato in it should be avoided

Foods to avoid

Other foods to avoid for proper healing are shellfish, junk food, fried foods, alcohol, pickled and smoked food, processed food, pastries, sodas and saturated fats. Which includes red meat in any form and no products with hydrogenated fat. Instead of cooking with butter or margarine, replace with olive oil

Tea Tree Oil

The use of tea tree as a treatment of psoriasis is as old as the hills. Tea tree oil comes from the leaves of Melaleuca tree, which is native to Australia. The oil is believed to have antiseptic properties. My grandmother believes tea tree works like an anesthetic, which calms infected areas while reducing the scratching. She told me that tea tree penetrates deeply into the skin, which helps diminish the scars caused by psoriasis. On further research I discovered that the oil helps remove dry and dead skin cells causing psoriasis. Applying the oil helps softening the plaques and clear psoriasis problem on the skin. It also contain a compound known as terpinen-4-ol which has potent anti-inflammatory property that helps you get relief from psoriasis. Below is the step by step guide to remedy psoriasis as learnt from my grandmother. I strongly recommend this band.

You need this:
- Tea tree oil
- Water
- Cotton ball

Directions:
- Pour few drops of tea tree oil into a bowl and add a reasonable amount of water into it.
- Stir the mixture properly and using the cotton ball soak a generous portion.
- Apply this to the affected areas and leave it to stay overnight.
- Wash off in the morning, pat dry your skin and apply your moisturizer of choice.

- Alternatively, you can use the combination of tea tree and olive oil. For this method, mix equal amount of tea tree and olive oil in a small bowl and warm the mixture for few minutes.
- Apply the warmed oil mixture on the affected areas of the skin. Leave it for a few moments to dry and then wash it off with water and pat dry the skin.

NB: Try as much as possible to use tea tree in its diluted form. For this remedy to work effectively, endeavor to use the best quality oil, which is cold pressed and organic.

Aloe Vera

I was dubbed the Aloe Vera specialist by my peers. We had aloe vera plants littered all over our backyard and am the only guy solely responsible for watering and catering for them. Aloe Vera was one of those remedies frequently used in my grandmother's herbal center. My grandmother believed that aloe vera was more effective in minimizing psoriasis severity more than any steroid cream. Like a good student, I kept a note book by my side, where I jotted down all she taught me. Although she died leaving all her research materials with me, which I promise to find the time to share most of her incredible works here with you. The aloe vera gel contains essential antioxidant and vitamins which help repair and restore damaged skin cells. The anti-inflammatory property helps soothes inflamed and irritated skin.

Direction:

Scrap out the gel from aloe vera and apply it directly on the infected skin. Leave it to dry, before washing it off. Repeat this process at least two times a day. Alternatively, drink aloe vera juice on an empty stomach early in the morning. If this poses a big deal for you, feel free to blend it with any non-citrus fruit. Another great alternative is to mix aloe vera with baking soda in 2:1 ratio. Apply this mixture on psoriasis and leave it for 10 minutes. Wash with clean water. Repeat this process once a daily.

Capsaicin

Capsaicin is the ingredient in chili peppers that make them hot. A study conducted on forty-four patients with symmetrically distributed psoriatic lesions, where capsaicin was applied to one side of their body and identical-appearing vehicle to the other side, shows that greater overall improvement was observed on sides treated with capsaicin compared to sides treated with vehicle. Researchers from the University Medical Center Freiburg, in Freiburg, Germany, found OTC creams containing capsaicin may help reduce the pain, inflammation, redness and scaling associated with psoriasis. Please note that this should be applied externally not taken internally

Oat Bath

Oat is considered to be one of nature's best skin soothers and helps calm and repair dry itchy and inflamed skin. My grandmother always advises her psoriasis patients to soak their selves in an oatmeal bath to relieve parched, rough, painful and sore skin. This singular practice also helps remove scales and calms redness

Directions:
- Pour 1/3 to ¾ cup of oatmeal into a bowl and press down the dry oatmeal with the back of your spoon. This is to get rid of any clump that might have formed in the storage.
- Gradually spoon the mixture into a coffee filter bag. Tie it off with a rubber band, string or ribbon. Fill you tub with relatively amount of hot water. Throw in the oatmeal in the back of the tub, away from the bath end with the running water. Allow to cool. As the tub cools to a tolerable temperature, the heat will cause the essences of oatmeal to disperse. Gently step into the tub when it is tepid, and gradually squeeze the oatmeal sachet to release more of the oatmeal liquid through the bath; be careful not to press too hard, to avoid breaking the sachet. Enjoy your bath and remember not to stay longer than 10 minutes

Vinegar Dip

This particular remedy is very useful; I have seen it work for a friend of mine living with psoriasis. Its disinfectant property helps soothe the minor burns and other. Hippocrates used vinegar to manage wounds. Vinegar help kill pathogens, including bacteria. It has traditionally been used for cleaning and disinfecting, treating nail fungus, lice, warts and ear infections.

You need:
- Apple cider vinegar
- Water
- Cotton Ball

Directions:
- Pour 1 cup of Apple cider vinegar into a reasonable amount of water to make a vinegar compress.
- Soak the cotton ball into the mixture and apply it directly on the plaques.
- Alternatively, you can apply it topically on the affected areas. You can as well mix two table spoon of ACV in a glass of water and drink it every night before going to bed.

Turmeric:

The active ingredient in turmeric is known as curcumin, which is a powerful antioxidant, used in the treatment of various skin diseases like skin cancer, psoriasis, scleroderma and tumors of the skin. Curcumin fights inflammation and protects the body from free radicals. Turmeric also improves collagen deposits and acts as a proangiogenic agent. There are various ways in which turmeric can be used in the treatment of psoriasis.

Included in your daily diet

Make a paste on turmeric powder and water: My friend Israel normally uses this method. He will mix the powder with a small amount of water or Vaseline and rub it on. I must warn you, doing this might cause tedious work in removing it. Everything you touch will turn yellow, and it hardly goes off. Sometimes it can take up to four days to come off; Israel can testify to this. To get around this, I suggest you buy powder with the dye removed; such as Indus Organic Turmeric or get extracts of pure curcumin.

Turmeric can be taken as a supplement. Not everybody is in love with turmeric, if you fall in this category do yourself a favor and go for turmeric supplements. You can as well make a tonic of turmeric powder and warm milk or with organic honey.

Castor Oil

Castor oil is one of the major oil in the treatment of psoriasis and can help moisturize the skin without any further irritation. Take few drops of castor oil and apply it directly on the affected areas. Leave it overnight. This will help reduce the intensity of psoriasis up to a certain extent. Please try not to apply this on cracked skin.

CHAPTER 36

Effective cures for Shingles

Shingles is not life-threatening, so don't be worried if you have one. I totally understand how painful it can be because I have been in that exact position in this past. I can still remember the painful blistering rash wrapped around my left torso – and the inflammation it caused me.

The symptoms are characterized by painful, burning sensation, red rash that starts a few days after the pain and fluid-filled blisters that break open and crust over. Most people often complain of fever, headache, fatigue and sensitivity to light, while for some, they experience the rash without pain. The good news is that shingles are not contagious, but it can still infect a person who hasn't had chickenpox in the past. Shingle and Chickenpox how are they related? Both are caused by the same virus (varicella-zoster) after recovering from chickenpox, the virus stays back and lies idle in your nerve tissue close to your spinal cord and brain. Years later the virus can be awakened by stress (emotional or physical). Thus, the disease is most common among individuals over the age of 50. Developing chicken pox at an early age may substantially lower the risk of developing shingles. I strongly advise you don't go the usual route of taking prescribed drug. I wouldn't dispute the fact that this drug works, but they sure do come with some adverse effects.

Effective Home Remedies for Shingles
Honey for Shingles

Honey works quite well in the treatment of shingles. This is partly because it draws fluid away from the wound and its high sugar content helps inhibit the growth of harmful microorganism.

You need
- High-quality Manuka Honey

Directions:
- The aim here is to keep the sores regularly bathed with honey. Apply honey in a semifluid form directly on the affected area.
- Do this four times daily.

An alternative is to try the mixture of honey and vinegar – make a paste of this combination and dab it on your sore. This is an effective way to make shingles dry up.

Baking Soda or Cornstarch

Applying baking soda to the rash helps dry the sores and make them heal quickly.

You need
- One tsp of baking soda
- Water

Directions:
Make a paste of baking soda and water by mixing a generous amount a baking soda with a small amount of water. Stir till you have a thick consistency. Apply this paste on the infected area as often as possible. This will help calm and dry the blisters.

Apple Cider Vinegar:

Apple Cider Vinegar is an excellent source of acetic acid which is a potent antimicrobial and can contribute to killing several type of bacteria.

You need:
- ½ cup Apple Cider Vinegar
- 2 cups of Distilled Water

Directions:
- Simply mix ½ of apple cider vinegar with 2 cups of water.
- Use a cotton swab to soak the mixture.
- Apply the swab to the affected areas.
- Repeat this 3 times daily. The shingles will gradually dry up.

Aloe Vera and Cayenne Pepper

This duo works very well in the treatment of shingles. Aloe Vera is well known for its soothing and healing effect, and it helps soothe the rash while pulling out moisture from it – this causes it to dry out and activate the healing process

You need:
- 2 tsp of aloe vera pulp
- Cayenne pepper

Directions:
- Using a teaspoon or knife, collect the pulp from the aloe vera.
- Mix the pulp with powdered cayenne pepper to form a consistent paste.
- Apply this paste on the affected area.
- Repeat this thrice daily, till the shingles dry up

Turmeric

Turmeric is another potent nature's ingredient for shingles. It can also be used for other skin infections like ringworm, bruise, leech, bites, inflammatory skin conditions, soreness inside of the mouth and infected wounds.

You need:
- 3 tsp of turmeric
- 3 cups of water

Directions:
- Bring 3 cups of water to boil, then add turmeric powder and allow it to form a paste.
- Apply the paste on affected areas. Repeat this twice daily. The shingles will begin to dry up

Use a Wet Compress.

Wet compress is usually used to reduce the inflammation resulting from shingles. Applying a wet compress of cold water will make you feel great while minimizing the itching.

You need:
- A wash cloth
- A bowl of cold water

Directions:
- Soak the washcloth in cold water, wring it out and apply it to affected area.
- Repeat this after several minutes to renew the feeling.
- Always remember to wash your towels after you use them on shingles.

Try Epsom Salt

Another remedy I strongly suggest you try out is the Epsom salt treatment. It works well in soothing inflammations and drying up the blisters.

You need:
- Three tsp of Epsom salt
- I glass of water

Directions:
Make a paste of Epsom salt by mixing it with a little amount of water. Apply the paste on the affected area. Repeat this twice daily as desired.

Use Calamine Lotion

I have found that Calamine lotion also works well in the soothing of inflammation and itching associated with Shingles. When applied to on affected area it evaporates from your skin while drawing moisture out of the blisters.

Garlic

Garlic has made its name as one of the strongest antiviral food, and it has proven to be great in the treatment of shingles.

Your need
- Five cloves of garlic

Directions:
- Simply make a paste of garlic by mashing five garlic cloves together.
- Apply the paste on affected area.
- Leave for about five minutes before washing off warm water.
- Repeat this few times daily for about two weeks.
- The shingles will gradually dry off. Garlic can also be eaten or taken orally. It is also available in capsules.

Oatmeal

Oatmeal bath and starch bath can also be used to heal irritated and painful skin.

You need:
- Oatmeal
- Luke warm water

Directions:
Stir a reasonable amount of oatmeal in lukewarm water. Hot water should be avoided, because they can further irritate your skin and worsen the rash. Immense yourself in the water and stay for at least 20 minutes. Then pat dry

Other Recommendations

- Those who have never had chickenpox or shingles before should avoid contact with those who have an outbreak of with both.
- Exposure to fluid from shingles causes chicken pox and possible shingles in near future.
- The varicella vaccine, although initially given to children as an immunization against chickenpox, can also be used for an adult who never had chicken pox – this reduces the chances and complications while minimizing the severity of the disease.

- Consumption of fresh vegetables like mushroom, yellow ball pepper, spinach, and tomato can help with the treatment of shingles. The best way to take these vegetables is through juicing.
- Try as much as possible to keep the inflamed skin clean and dry
- Do not pick the blisters
- Do not share any clothes or towels with others.
- Lemon balm and coconut oil can also be used to treat shingles

CHAPTER 37

Amazing uses of Turmeric as First Aid

While in India, Mrs. Aishwarya, the lady I stayed with during my stay India, taught me the several uses of turmeric. On a particular occasion, her daughter Amita slit her fingers while slicing bitter gourd. The bleeding was heavy and in my mind, I thought the best solution was to get her to the hospital.

Mrs. Aishwarya, on getting to the scene didn't panic at all. She told everyone to step aside and turned to me said "daro mat , har baat ke niyantran mein hai" which meant I shouldn't panic, everything was under control. She cleaned the surface with water – after which she applied turmeric powder to cover the wounded surface. After a few days, the turmeric congealed with the blood and fell off. She reapplied it again after cleaning the wound. Turmeric owes this ability to its anti-inflammatory, antibiotic and natural healing properties.

Mrs. Aishwarya also told me that turmeric can also be used to soothe insect and scorpion sting. She said that a week earlier, before my arrival, an unknown species of scorpion stringed her husband – the poor guys started vomiting, blood pressure was going high, and his heart beat accelerated, and he cried like a kid. She applied a thick paste of turmeric over the bite, which acted as an antidote to the poison and controlled the inflammation. Swelling due to sprain can also be remedied by turmeric. Just apply it topically over the area or take it internally.

Mrs. Aishwarya prepares the lemon, honey and turmeric cleanse. The cleanse is extremely effective in getting rid of toxins from the body. It's a most drink for the whole family every morning. To prepare yours, make available the ingredients: lemon juice, 1/4 tsp of turmeric and a glass if warm water. The preparation is very simple, just combine all the ingredients in warm water and stir well. To be taken before breakfast.

Turmeric for Skin Problems:

In India, the use of Turmeric for skins problem is as old as the hills. It's a part of the ancient Ayurveda treatment for skin related problems. To heal skin infection like eczema, mix 10 grams of turmeric, 50 grams of neem powder and butter together. Apply this paste on the affected area. This will help reduce the itching while providing a cooling effect. Neem and turmeric are well known in India for getting rid of itching. Turmeric can also be mix with butter alone and applied to eczema and itching skin. Taking turmeric orally is also recommended. Do this every morning and evening

Depression:

Everyone gets depressed once in a while in their lives. Some have become so used to it; that it's a normal lifestyle for them. I can't keep count of how many times I went into depression while writing this book. If you are reading this book them, know that I have conquered my fears. Other factors like hormone imbalance, genetic changes, stressful life situations and medical problems like cardiovascular diseases, strokes and diabetes can substantially contribute to depression. Most people has resulted to using anti-depressant drugs like Tricyclic antidepressant, Serotonin-norepinephrine reuptake inhibitors. These drugs are not without side effect. If there is one thing that helped me combat my depression, it is turmeric. Researchers from the Government Medical College (Bhavnagar, Gujarat, India) published the results to evaluate curcumin's ability to manage depression in a controlled setting. They took 60 volunteers diagnosed with the major depressive disorder. They were divided into three groups to determine how patients treated by curcumin compared against fluoxetine (Prozac) and a combination of the two reacted. It was discovered that the principal curcuminoid in turmeric is not only as effective as Prozac in managing depression, but it also doesn't carry with it all the dangerous side effects as anti-depressive drugs do. Curcumin protects you against depression in 3 ways. Firstly by acting against oxidative and inflammatory responses generated during a depression. It modulates the levels of neurotransmitter in the brain and also increases the amount of neurotrophic factors which are responsible for the growth and survival of nerve cells

Get this
- 8 cups distilled water
- Three tablespoons pure turmeric powder or 1 1/2 cups peeled and sliced fresh turmeric
- 2 cup distilled water (if using fresh turmeric)

Procedure (if using powder):
- Bring 8 cups water to boil.
- Add turmeric powder and bring the temperature down to a slow simmer for 12 minutes.
- Allow it to cool.
- Strain through a fine muslin cloth.
- Store in a clean dry glass jar and refrigerate.

While using fresh turmeric, put on a latex food grade gloves. Peel and finely slice turmeric until you have 2 cups. Throw in the turmeric into boiling water and let it simmer for about 15 – 18 minutes. Strain through a fine muslin cloth. Then store in a clean, dry glass jar and put in a refrigerator.

Turmeric for diabetes

It will surprise you that this powerful spice has a powerful therapeutic intervention for type 2 diabetics. Various studies have confirmed its effectiveness in reducing blood sugar and reversing insulin resistance. But take caution to avoid turmeric supplement if you are already using any hyperglycemia medication to treat diabetics, although both the drugs can reduce blood sugar but can also cause immense complications. To take it even further and prove the effectiveness of turmeric in the treatment of diabetics. A Particular study in the Auburn University revealed that curcumin suppresses glucose production in the liver and it is 400 times more potent than Metformin (a common diabetes drug) in the activation of AMPK and its downstream target acetyl-CoA carboxylase (ACC). Another study conducted in the central food technological research Institute, Mysore, Indian also proved that curcumin can help bring down the high lipid levels in diabetic animals. This was tested by giving 0.5% curcumin supplement to drug induced diabetic rat for eight weeks. The result was that their blood cholesterol levels dropped significantly. Turmeric also acts as an anti-diabetic and antioxidant in diabetes in type 1 diabetes – also improve metabolic function and reduce the risk of plaque buildup in the arteries of type 2 diabetes patients.

Turmeric for Asthma

Turmeric is an excellent herb for asthma – its anti-inflammatory property helps clear mucus in your lungs and soothes the irritation and inflammation caused due to airways blockage. The allergic response is triggered when T-lymphocytes from your immune system release a particular compound that causes inflammation and irritation. Researchers have found that turmeric can block the release of these inflammation-causing compound. It also helps dilate the blood vessels that allows for a better flow of air, restores normal breathing patterns, relaxes the muscle spasms, thins out the blood and gives relief from the asthmatic inflammation which causes swelling in the lungs and trouble breathing. To use turmeric take three grams of turmeric powder and mix it with 7 grains of black pepper. Mix this with pure mustard oil and lick this paste early in the morning. You can also stir 1 teaspoon of turmeric powder in a glass of water and drink this thrice a day.

Turmeric is also available in capsules, pills or tincture. If you are lactose intolerant simply mix the following ingredients, ¼ teaspoon of turmeric powder, ½ teaspoon grated ginger and ¼ teaspoon of pepper. Add this mixture into a little pot of water and bring it to boil. Pour this into an empty glass and allow it to cool for a few minutes before drinking.

Rheumatoid Arthritis

Numerous studies conducted on turmeric has proven its anti-inflammatory properties and its ability to modify immune system responses. A particular study conducted in 2006 showed that Turmeric is very effective in preventing joint inflammation then reducing joint inflammation. Another clinical trial undertaken in 2010 found that a turmeric supplement called Meriva provided long-term improvement in pain and function in 100 patients. The best way for Rheumatoid Arthritis patients to take turmeric is to take it as a part of their diet. They can also go for supplements when there is no other choice. Its 100% save to take up to 1 gm of turmeric powder.

Cancer

A 2011 study conducted by the University of Texas MD Anderson Cancer Center, researchers revealed that the curcumin extract differentiates between cancer cells and normal cells while activating cancer cell death. Studies have shown that curcumin, the active ingredient in turmeric helps in several forms of cancer, including breast, stomach, lung, liver and colon cancer. It inhibits the growth of cancer cells, boost antioxidant levels and the immune system - while killing the cancer cells.

Lab results have found curcumin proficient in:

- Killing large cell B-cell lymphoma cells (the most common reason for non-Hodgkin lymphoma).
- Inhibiting an enzyme (COX-2) that causes adverse inflammation, which can lead to cancer.
- Impeding vascular epithelial growth (a polypeptide that stimulates new blood supply) to starve cancer cells of their oxygen and fuel source.
- Inducing a tumor suppressor gene.
- Stopping metastasis (spread from one organ to another) of cancer cells.
- Preventing regrowth of cancer stem cells.

Brain Health and Memory

Turmeric is extremely healing for the brain and for increasing memory function. A particular animal research found a bioactive compound in turmeric called aromatic-turmerone which is shown to help increase neural stem cell growth in the brain by as much as 80 percent at certain concentrations. Neural stem cells differentiate into neurons and play a significant role in self-repair. The research also reveals that aromatic-turmerone also helps in the recovery of brain function in neurodegenerative diseases such as stroke and Alzheimer. Also, researchers at the Institute of Neuroscience and Medicine in Julich, Germany, studied the effects of aromatic-turmerone by injecting rats with the compound. After which their brains were scanned. It revealed that a particular part the brain involved in nerve cell growth became more active after the injection.

Stomach Disorders:

It's always handy to have turmeric around the house. You will appreciate it more when you have any stomach disorder. Turmeric can be used to give instant relief to most stomach problems. For instance, if you are suffering from stomach pain, boil 10gms of the bark of turmeric root in about quarter a liter of water. Drink the resulting solution for instant relief. Turmeric is also a great cure for diarrhea. Simply mix ½ tsp of turmeric powder in water. Take this portion three times daily for immediate relief. Or you can grind an equal amount of turmeric and ginger roots to make 2-5 gms of the powdered mixture, pour it into a glass of boiling water, let it simmer. Drink the resulting solution. I have also found that taking ten gms of turmeric with a cup of plain yogurt also helps in the treatment of diarrhea and dysentery. This is due to turmeric powerful anti-microbial agent.

Turmeric for Urinary

Turmeric contains a naturally occurring substance known as curcumin, which is effective in killing a variety of strains of strain bacteria and treatment of urinary tract infection – its antioxidant property boosts the activity of the immune system and prevents damage to the kidney. In turn, fastens the healing process as well as prevents the recurring infections. According to a 2009 article published in the journal "Food Chemistry" found that the antibacterial action of curcumin was effective in killing both Staphylococcus aureus and E. coli bacteria, which commonly causes UTI. Turmeric also helps in the treatment of kidney disease; it does this by improving the activities of glutathione peroxidase which aids in the reduction of free radical generation by curbing the lipid peroxidation process in kidney microsomes and mitochondria. To remedy watery urination with excessive discharge and foul smell, take one gram each of turmeric and sesame and 2 grams of jaggery. This should be taken with boiled and then cooled water in morning and evening for a few days.

Turmeric for teeth whitening

I swear this work all the time, and I have seen it work for a whole lot of other people. As counter-intuitive as it might seem, turmeric is used to whiten the teeth. After I discovered this, I hardly use toothpaste again. I wish I can show you how white this has made my teeth. I still have lots of turmeric powder I brought from India. To whiten your teeth with turmeric, wet your toothbrush and dip it into 1/8 teaspoon of turmeric powder. Now, brush your teeth the standard way. Instead of rinsing off afterward, just allow the turmeric to sit on your teeth for about 3-5 minutes. Then spit out and rinse thoroughly. I usually compliment the first turmeric brushing with a second brushing with baking soda for an extra whitening.

Turmeric for scalp

A friend of mine gave me this little secret; I didn't find it hard to believe, because she is a living testimony of someone who rocks her natural hair. She told that combining a mixture of turmeric and olive oil - using it on your scalp can help get rid of dandruff and improve your overall scalp condition. If you don't have olive oil, use jojoba or coconut oil. Massage it into your scalp, leave for 15 minutes then wash off.

Liver Diseases

A particular research conducted at the Saint Louis University in Missouri proved that curcumin present in turmeric helps prevent and treat fatty liver disease. The study also reveals that curcumin reduced the effect of leptin that harms the liver cells while preventing the development of liver damage from nonalcoholic steatohepatitis. Another study evaluated the effect of turmeric on the livers of rat and found that turmeric prevented the formation of the inflammatory chemical known as cyclooxygenase-2 (COX-2) and boosted the formation of liver detoxification enzymes, including one called gluthianone S-transferase and also inhibited free radical damage. Turmeric shares similar liver protectant compounds that milk thistle and artichoke leaves contain. It is said to shrink engorged hepatic ducts, so it can be useful to treat liver conditions such as hepatitis, cirrhosis, and jaundice.

Skin and Aging

Turmeric has many healing properties for the skin. It possesses several biological properties that aids in combating signs of aging. It reduces inflammation and redness while promoting skin healing. Due to its antioxidant properties it is widely used for rejuvenating the skin. It helps soften lines and wrinkles while giving the face a more youthful glow. It is also very useful with rosacea. It's antibacterial and is great for blemishes acne and skin balance. Turmeric is excellent for improving the texture of the skin because it is an exfoliant but also rich in antioxidants.

Here's a recipe for a homemade turmeric facial mask:

Ingredients
- One teaspoon of turmeric
- yogurt teaspoon of raw organic honey
- One teaspoon of milk (or natural yoghurt)

To prepare this mask, start by putting turmeric into a little bowl – then add honey and plain yogurt. Make sure it forms a thick paste that can sit on your face. Cover your clothes properly because turmeric is a dye and can stain anything it comes in touches. Apply the mask on your face and massage evenly. Turmeric is also anti-inflammatory and can help reduce darks circles under eyes. Leave the mask on your face for about 20 minutes and then wash off with cool water and pat dry.

CHAPTER 38

An Abscessed Tooth? Here are the remedies

An abscessed tooth is a common term used to describe an infection at the root of a tooth or an infection that occurs between the gum and a tooth.

An abscessed tooth causes severe tooth decay and can be caused by bacteria that enters the tooth through a dental cavity, chip or crack. It spreads all the way down to the root tip and can further cause severe pain and inflammation. The affected tooth loses its ability to combat infections, which then reaches the pulp chamber of the tooth. When the pulp in the root tooth dies, this decreases the pain. While this doesn't mean the infection has healed, as it will continue to spread and destroy the tissues. If left untreated, it may spread to the bone that supports the tooth and can cause severe, life-threatening complications. Gingivitis can also cause an abscessed tooth. Other factors include severe tooth decay, poor dental hygiene, high sugar diet and sticky foods.

The symptom of the abscessed tooth includes, throbbing and sharp toothache, pain when chewing food, change in taste senses, bad breath, swelling of the cheek, red and sore gums, difficulty in swallowing food, swollen lymph nodes under your jaw, fever, change in taste senses and general discomfort.

Below are the amazing home remedies for abscessed tooth

Water and Salt Rinse

This a popular solution that even your dentist will recommend. Salt has antiseptic and antibacterial properties that can help reduce inflammation, prevent the growth of bacteria in the mouth and stop any further infections.

You need:
- ½tsp of salt
- 1 glass of warm water

Directions
- Pour the salt into warm water and mix thoroughly. Use the mixture to rinse your mouth thoroughly then spit out. Repeat this 3-4 time daily to clear infections and reduce discomfort and pain

Oil Pulling

The use of oil pulling as a remedy for tooth infection is as old as the hills. It is widely used in ancient Ayurveda practice and also in the treatment of abscessed tooth or painful gums. Oil pulling helps reduce the number of bacterias and toxins from the mouth and also promotes the overall oral health.

You need:
- 1 tbsp of coconut oil
- Warm water

Directions
- Pour one teaspoon of extra-virgin coconut oil in your mouth and swishing the oil inside your mouth for about 15 minutes and spit the oil out. Rinse your mouth thoroughly with warm water. Repeat this twice daily especially in the morning on an empty stomach for about a month

Garlic

Garlic contains an active compound called allicin, which is a natural antibiotic that helps prevent the bacterial infections of abscess tooth. It also has anti-inflammatory properties which give relief from swelling and pain.

Material Needed
- Garlic Cloves 3-4

Direction
- Peel and wash the cloves properly, then crush them and squeeze out the juice, which releases the compound allicin, apply the juice to your abscess tooth. Repeat this process at least 2 times daily
- Alternatively, eat 2-3 cloves of garlic (chew properly to release the allicin)

Wet Black Tea Bag

Black tea bag contains antioxidant that helps fight infections and promote good oral health. It is highly helpful in dental abscesses by bringing the infection to the head and absorbing some of the toxins/pus.

Materials needed
- Warm water
- Black tea bag

Directions
- Soak the black tea bag in warm water for a few minutes. Wring it out and place on the swollen area while holding or sucking on it. Leave it there for few hours or overnight and rinse your mouth with salt-water solution afterward. Repeat once daily for a couple of weeks

Hydrogen Peroxide

Hydrogen Peroxide is an excellent antimicrobial agent that can help get rid of tooth abscess. It has a disinfectant and antibacterial property that helps kill the bacteria that causes abscessed tooth, thereby reducing inflammation and pain.

Materials Needed
- Two tsp of Hydrogen Peroxide
- One tsp of warm water
- Baking soda

- Cotton ball (optional)

Directions
- Mix 2 teaspoon of hydrogen peroxide with one tables spoon of warm water. Use this mixture to rinse your mouth thoroughly, and spit out
- Alternatively, mix one teaspoon of baking soda with two teaspoons of hydrogen peroxide to make a paste. Apply this paste on the affected areas for a few minutes and rinse your mouth thoroughly with warm water. Do this for a couple of weeks.

Apple Cider Vinegar

Apple cider vinegar is another very effective home remedy for an abscessed tooth. It contains two beneficial acids called acetic acid and malic acid, which are excellent antibacterial, antimicrobial and anti-fungal properties. It also has disinfectant and inflammatory properties that help reduce pain and inflammation while disinfecting the area.

Materials
- One tablespoon Apple Cider Vinegar

Directions
- Pour apple cider vinegar in your mouth and swish it thoroughly. Leave it for 5 minutes and spit it out. Rinse your mouth properly with warm water. Repeat this 2-4 times daily for a month

Turmeric

Turmeric is well used to reduce inflammation caused by an abscessed tooth. It is rich in antibiotic, antiseptic and anti-inflammatory properties and also helps promotes oral health

Materials:
- Warm water
- One tsp turmeric powder

Directions:
- Mix 1 teaspoon of turmeric powder with a little water to make a paste of it. Apply the paste directly on the affected tooth. Allow it to sit for about 15minutes, then rinse off.
- Alternatively, mix 14 teaspoons of turmeric with one teaspoon of olive oil. Apply the paste to the affected area. Allow to sit for 15 minutes, then rinse off

Oregano Oil

Oregano oil contains antibacterial, antioxidant and antimicrobial properties which help remove infections. When used on an abscessed tooth, numbs the area - this makes the pain seize instantly. Oregano oil is widely used for abscessed tooth because it helps abscess drainage while killing the bacteria in the pus. It also boosts immunity and helps fight tooth infections and speeds up healing process.

Materials Needed
- 2-3 drops off oregano oil
- Cotton swab

Do this
- Pour a few drops of oregano oil directly on the cotton swab. Apply the swab directly on the affected tooth and leave to stay for about 5 minutes.
- Alternatively, prepare a mouthwash by mixing 3 to 5 drops of oregano with ¼ cup of warm water. Use the mixture to swish your mouth for about 5 minutes and spit out the mixture. Repeat this remedies for about 3 or 4 times daily

Peppermint Oil

Peppermint is a potent treatment for an abscessed tooth. Its antibacterial and anti-inflammatory properties help reduce inflammation and relieve you of the pain associated with the abscessed tooth.

Materials Needed
- 2-4 drops of Peppermint oil
- Cotton swab

Directions
- Pour few drops of peppermint oil on the swab and apply directly to the affected area. Hold the swab against your tooth for a few minutes before letting go. Alternatively, you can use your finger to apply the oil gently on the affected tooth. Repeat this process 3-4 times a day for at least a month.

Potato

Potato has antiseptic properties, and it's alkaline in nature with acidic properties. Its acidic property is said to help slough off dead cells and other toxins.

Materials
- Slice of raw potato

Directions
- Take the slice of raw potato and place it in affected areas. Leave it there to sit for 30 minutes or leave overnight. Then remove the potato. You should notice a bit of discolouration over it; this is due to the toxins pulled out of the infected tooth.

Chamomile

Chamomile contains anti-inflammatory properties which can heal injured tissues. It comes in herbs and tea form; both can be used to remedy abscessed tooth.

Directions
- Drink 3 to 4 cups of chamomile tea daily
- To soothe swelling, make a poultice of chamomile and apply it topically over affected area several times a day
- Alternatively, wet the tea bag and hold it against the infected tooth.

Echinacea

Echinacea is widely considered a natural antibiotic and it helps relieve pain and inflammation caused by infections. Echinacea is available in tinctures and capsules
.
Materials
- Echinacea herb
- One tsp tea bag
- Water

Directions
- Mix warm water with the herb or teabag. Leave it to steep for about 5 minutes, then strain the mixture. Use the mixture to rinse your mouth thoroughly. Repeat this 2-3 times daily

Additional Tips

To prevent abscessed tooth, below are a few tips to bear in mind
- Always brush your teeth twice daily.
- You can apply cold compress on your cheek near the affected area to get a painrelief.

- Make sure you always use toothbrush containing fluoride.
- Use an antimicrobial mouthwash to swish your mouth every morning after brushing your teeth.
- Endeavor to change your toothbrush every 3 to 4 months.
- Quit smoking and the use of tobacco.
- Chewing too much of gum should be avoided
- Avoid junk food and eats healthy foods.
- When suffering from tooth pain or infection avoid caffeine.

CHAPTER 39

Effective treatment for Asthma

Asthma was derived from the Greek term "breathlessness" A feeling of not being able to get enough air, no matter how hard the victims tries. The typical symptoms are abnormal breathing sounds, coughing and wheezing, a feeling of tightness in the chest and difficulty in breathing. During this attack, spasms in the muscles surrounding the bronchi constricts, impeding the outward passage of air. Asthma is of two forms: allergic and non-allergic.

Both often occurs together. The reason why people develop asthma is still unknown although in some cases, it is heredity. What triggers asthma is different from person to persons. But in most cases it includes exposure to toxic chemicals, exposure to allergens, exposure to cold air and emotional upset.

Magnesium Supplement

The mineral found in magnesium acts as a bronchodilator, which means that it relaxes and open the bronchial tract - the air way to the lungs that becomes constricted during asthma attacks.

- Take a daily 500-milligram supplement of magnesium aspartate or magnesium citrate. This supplement should be taken daily, for six months.

Boswellia

Boswellia plays a huge role in reducing leukotrienes, which causes bronchial muscles to contract. A particular study shows that patients who took boswellia experienced decreased asthma symptoms and asthma indicators.

Mullein Oil

Mullein Oil is a well-known remedy for bronchial congestion. It has a soothing effect on bronchial passage. The oil stops coughs, unclogs bronchial tubes and help clear up asthma attacks.
It can be taken in tea or fruit juice

- Add a few peeled garlic cloves into the oil and take a few sip

Mustard Oil

Mustard oil comes in handy during asthma attacks.

- Rub some brown mustard oil on your chest and massage thoroughly for instant relief
- Alternatively, heat some mustard oil with a little camphor, then pour it into a bowl, when it cools down, gently rub it on your chest and upper back, till symptoms subside.
- Mix 1/4 teaspoon of mustard and pippal (or black pepper) together, put the mixture in a cup of hot water and add two teaspoons of honey. Drink 2 to 3 times daily
- Mix a teaspoon of brown mustard oil with one teaspoon of organic sugar. Take a dose of this mixture twice daily on an empty stomach

Ginger

Ginger is a well-known remedy for asthma due to it a potent antioxidant activity which constitutes of gingerols, shogaols, and zingerones. These compounds have anti-inflammatory and analgesic properties similar to non-steroidal anti-inflammatory drugs. Ginger enhances bronchodilation, a substance that dilates the bronchi and bronchioles, decreasing resistance in the respiratory airway and increasing airflow to the lungs.

- Mix one teaspoon of ground ginger with half cup of water and take one tablespoon of this mixture before bedtime.
- Add small pieces of ginger into a pot of boiling water. Let it steep for five minutes, allow to cool down and then drink the mixture
- Mix ginger juice with pomegranate juice and honey. Drink one tablespoon two or three times a day
- Boil one tablespoon of fenugreek seed in a cup of water. Pure one teaspoon of ginger juice and honey into it and mix thoroughly. Drink this solution every morning and evening.
- You can as well eat the ginger raw

Garlic

Garlic has anti-inflammatory properties, which makes it a good remedy for asthma. The below garlic treatment can help clear congestion in your lungs during the early stages of asthma.
- Boil two or three cloves in one-quarter cup of milk. Allow it to cool to room temperature and drink up.

Nettle Tea

The herb contains a form of histamine which helps control allergic reactions. Their antihistamine properties help control sneezing and itching caused by asthma attacks. Nettle tea cuts the phlegm and congestion that blocks the airway. It is available in root, leaf and powdered forms.

Figs

Fig plays a vital role in reducing the various symptoms of asthma attack. The nutritional content in figs helps promote respiratory health and helps drain phlegm and alleviate breathing difficulties.

- Clean 3-4 dry figs and soak them in warm water overnight. Eat the soaked figs and drink the fig water on an empty stomach. Repeat this remedy for a few months

Honey

Honey is known as one of the oldest natural remedies for asthma due to the alcohol and ethereal oil in it

- Inhaling the smell of honey during crisis produces positive results for some victims
- Mix one teaspoon of honey with on-half of cinnamon powder and drink before bedtime. This remedy helps remove phlegm from your throat and allow you to sleep well

Onions

The sulfur content of onion helps decrease inflammation in the lungs, and its anti-inflammatory properties help reduce constriction in the airways for asthma patients

- Cut some pieces of onion and chew it, to clear your air passage

Rosemary Tea.

Rosemary is rich in the antioxidant polyphenol and helps reduce airway inflammation in children with asthma. It can also be used to make tea due to its asthma-fighting properties

- Add one teaspoon of rosemary to eight ounces of water, boil the mixture and steep it for five minutes. Add honey and lemon. Drink the mixture before bed time

Lemon

Lemon is high in vitamin C and rich in antioxidants which can greatly reduce asthma symptoms and should be drank by asthma patient to reduce asthma attacks. Lemon also helps kill the germs which are present in the mucus underlining the air vessel.

- Dilute the lemon juice in one glass of water. Drink this mixture during meals.
- Alternatively dilute the juice of 1 lemon in a glass of distilled water and add sugar to it.

Safflower Seeds

The safflower acts as an expectorant and helps reduce spasm by making the firmed sputum or mucus in your airway soft so that it can be expelled to give you needed relief.

- Mix the safflower seed powder with honey. Take this mixture 1-2 times daily
Take precaution:

Safflower may slow down blood clotting, so if you have a bleeding problem, avoid using safflower seeds.

Licorice

Licorice root is anti-inflammatory and has been used successfully for thousands of years to relieve asthma symptoms and breathing difficulties caused by several short-term respiratory illnesses. It soothes swollen airways, inhibits histamine release, helps loosen mucus and airways. Licorice root also aids in the relaxation of bronchial spasms and relieves soreness and tightness in the throat. Licorice also comes in oil form.

- Add 20 to 40 drops of licorice tincture to a cup of water and let it cool to room temperature, before drinking

Steam Inhalation

Steam inhalation is required when you have asthma cough because it prevents the phlegm that is trapped inside from thickening and causing asthma.

- Boil adequate amount of water and cover your head with a thick towel while inhaling the steam.
- Alternatively, add a few drops of eucalyptus oil or peppermint oil to relieving the airways of the phlegm. The hot steam will cause you to cough up the mucus, and your nose will start running well again

CHAPTER 40

Banish Acne with these simple remedies

According to Mayo Clinic, Acne is a skin condition that occurs when your hair follicles become plugged with oil and dead skin cells. Living with Acne can be frustrating and most times we fall prey to several store bought creams with promises of Acne treatment; which does nothing but cause more harm than good.

Acne occurs when the pores on your skin become blocked with oil, dead skin, or bacteria. Each pore on your skin is the opening to a follicle. The follicle is made up of a hair and a sebaceous (oil) gland. The oil gland releases sebum (oil), which travels up the hair, out of the pore, and onto your skin. I have found that a combination of a few home remedies can help treat acne.

Below are a few that works best with Acne:

Baking Soda

Baking soda works well for acne; I can guarantee you that. Baking soda is the remedy my sisters use to treat acne. It works for skin exfoliation and helps remove dead skin. It is also antiseptic and anti-inflammatory.

Get this
- One tsp of baking soda
- Little water

Directions
- Make a paste of baking soda by adding a small amount of water to it. Gently massage your face with this paste. With more emphasis on the acne. Leave the dough to sit for about 5 minutes. Wash off with Luke warm water. Repeat this process for two or three times a week

- Alternatively, you create a reasonable mixture of baking soda, cinnamon powder, lemon juice and honey. Massage the mixture on your face, leave it to sit for least 5 minutes. Then rinse off.

Tea Tree

It might sound ironic that am asking you to use tea tree to remedy acne. When it's a known fact that excessive oil in your pores can lead to acne. Tea tree is not like other oils. It is more of a solvent oil that cuts through the dead skin and extra sebum while unblocking your pores. Tea tree is well known as one of the best remedies for acne and has amazing antiseptic, antibacterial, antifungal and antiviral properties which help to kill the bacteria causing the acne. It can also be used in the healing of hypertrophic scars. When the case is acne, fear no more, go for tea tree

Get this
- Tea tree oil
- Warm water
- Cotton balls

Directions

- Dilute your tea tree oil in water (1 part oil to 9 part water). Soak the cotton bud into the mixture and apply on affected areas. Repeat this process three times daily. Always remember to dilute your tea tree before using. The reason for diluting tea tree is because it's too concentrated for the skin to handle.
- Some people may be allergic to tea tree, so before using it, test a drop of it in any part of your body. Leave it to sit for hours. If you experience any rashes, you may be allergic to it. So it's best not to put it on your face

Lemon

Lemon is an effective remedy for acne. It's a natural disinfectant which helps kill the bacteria that cause acne. When applied to the face, it helps clean out the dirt accumulated in the pores while hardening the sebum.

You need

- Lemon
- Cotton swab

Directions

- Squeeze out the juice from the lemon into a small bowl. Dab your cotton bud into the small bowl. Clean up your face with warm water and dry with a clean towel. With the soaked cotton swab, dab it on the acne and leave the lemon juice to sit on the acne for about 30 minutes. Then rinse the face thoroughly.
- Make sure to wash off before going under-the-sun to avoid the bleaching effect on the face. If you have chosen to implement this remedy at night. You can leave the lemon juice to sit on your face overnight.

Honey

Honey is an excellent choice for acne treatment; it contains lots of antioxidant and vitamins like vitamin B2, B3, and B5 as well as other minerals. It is also a natural antibiotic, anti-inflammatory and moisturizing agent. Honey helps fight off the bacteria that causes acne and also heal wound associated with acne. It owes this its ability to heal wound to its natural hydrogen peroxide produced in honey by the enzyme glucose oxidase. Experts consider Manuka honey and raw honey, to be the two best forms of honey for acne treatment

You need

- Raw honey (Unprocessed or even Manuka honey)
- Cotton ball or pad (optional)
- Warm water

Directions:

- Take a reasonable amount of honey using your finger or cotton ball. Apply the honey to your acne or all over your face. Leave it to sit for at least 30 minutes. Wash off with warm water. Repeat this twice weekly for best results.
- You could also add about 1/2 teaspoon of cinnamon to your honey, to its antibacterial properties.

Toothpaste

It will amaze you that, the toothpaste lying around your bathroom is a remedy for acne.

You need

- Toothpaste

Directions

- Apply a small amount of white toothpaste on the acne. Leave it to sit overnight. The toothpaste helps reduce the swelling while drying out the acne. Repeat this three times weekly. You should begin to see improvement after the end of one week

Oatmeal

Oatmeal is another great remedy you should consider trying out. Oatmeal works by cleansing the skin pores and absorbing excess oil while exfoliating the skin. When used as a mask, they reduce inflammation and redness that accompanies breakouts.

Get this

- One serving of oatmeal
- Lemon
- Water
- Two tablespoons raw honey

Directions

- Mix one teaspoon of honey and the juice of half a lemon in a cup of cooked oatmeal. Rub this mixture over the affected areas or the entire face. Let it sit for about 30 minutes. Then rinse off with lukewarm water. Repeat this twice ever week to see the result.

loe Vera

The anti-inflammatory and soothing properties of Aloe Vera can help treat acne. The herb also helps regenerate damaged tissues, therefore, boosting the healing process.

You need
• Aloe Vera

Directions
• Scrap out the gel contained inside the aloe vera. Gently apply the gel on the affected areas. Leave it for at least one hour and wash off afterward. Repeat this twice daily. This remedy will also make your skin glow and become lighter.

Turmeric

Turmeric is another powerful remedy for acne. When applied in a paste form on the acne destroys the Propionibacterium that causes inflammation and also helps reduce excess oil from the skin. Turmeric is rich in anti-oxidant and anti-inflammatory properties which are both beneficial in the treatment of acne.

You need
• ¼ teaspoon of powdered turmeric
• Two teaspoons of coconut oil

Directions
• Make a paste of turmeric by mixing up a ¼ teaspoon of powdered turmeric to 2 teaspoons of coconut oil. Stir the mixture thoroughly. Spread the mixture evenly on your face. Let it sit for at least 15 minutes. Rinse out with warm water. Do not leave overnight, because turmeric can stain the skin.
• Alternatively, you can mix eight tablespoons turmeric powder mixed with five tablespoons olive oil or sesame oil to make a paste of it.

Apple Cider Vinegar

The use of harsh cleanser and soap can disrupt our skins natural acid mantle, which is needed to protect the skin against germs, bacteria, and pollution. Apple cider vinegar helps restore the skin's acid mantle and balances your skin pH, leading to fewer blemishes and more even tone. It also kills bacteria, removes excess dirt, oil, and dead skin.

You need

- Apple cider vinegar
- Glass of water
- Cotton Swab

Directions

Pour in a small amount of apple cider vinegar into a glass and add a reasonable amount of water into it. The ratio of water depends on how sensitive your skin is. A ratio of one part apple cider vinegar to two or three part water is most common. Use the cotton swab to soak a reasonable amount of the diluted apple cider vinegar and apply to skin. Wait until the toner has dried and then use whatever other lotions, potions and creams you wish. Do this twice a day or anytime you wash your face, for best results.

Raw Tomatoes

Tomatoes are rich in antioxidants and vitamins A and C. They helps tighten the skin pore and shrink pimples

You will need

- Raw Tomatoes (one will be enough)

Directions

- Slice the tomato and rub the open half on the acne affected areas. Massage your skin with the tomatoes for a few seconds. Rinse off with warm water afterward. Repeat this twice daily for best results.
- Alternatively, mix up the juice from cucumber, avocados, and tomatoes. Apply the mixture on your face. Leave it to sit for 15-20 minutes before washing off with water.

Egg White

I got this remedy from a reliable source on the web. Egg white helps tighten up the surface of the skin and reduce the size of the pores; mostly used as a remedy for discoloration caused my acne.

You need

- 2 Eggs

Directions

- Separate the egg yolk from the whites. Add one tablespoon of lemon juice to the mix (to help loosen blackheads and whiteheads). Whisk the egg until it becomes a foam. Apply this evenly on your face, while massaging the face. Leave it to sit for about 15 minutes. Rinse off and moisturize your skin.

Papaya for a pimple prone

Papaya is another excellent remedy for acne. A friend revealed the treatment to me. He used it and recorded great results, so it worth trying out. Papaya does this by removing dead skin cells and excess lips from the surface of the skin, thereby leaving it soft and smooth. It also contains an enzyme, papain, which helps reduce inflammation and prevents pus from forming.

Get this

- One fresh papaya

Directions

- Make a paste of papaya; you can do this with your blender. Wash your face properly and apply the mashed papaya to your skin. Leave it to sit for 20 minutes. Rinse your face with warm water and moisturize your face.

Orange Peels

As much as this surprises you to know, it works. When I discovered that white inner orange peel is edible and contains more vitamin C. A, I marveled. Orange peel can help ward off bacteria and extra oil/dead skin cells clogging up the pores in your skin. It owes this to its citric acid, vitamin C, and astringent properties. The peel, as well as the juice, can be used.

Get this.

- 2 Orange peels
- Clean, fresh water

Directions

- Spread your fresh orange peels under the sun and leave it to dry out completely. Grind the dried peel into a powder form and add a little water (don't make it too watery), to turn it into a paste. Apply the paste to acne areas and leave it to sit for about 15 minutes. Wash off your face with warm water and use your moisturizer

Potato Acne Remedy

Potato is rich in potassium, sulfur, phosphorus and chloride, all of which are beneficial to remedy blemishes. They are also heavy on antioxidant that helps the growth of new skin cells.

Get this

- 1 potato

Directions

- Cut the potato into rounded slices. Rub the slice gently on your face in a circular motion. Keep doing this till the slice feels dry. Repeat the same process with another slice, do this for about 20 minutes. Leave the potato juice to sit for about 15-20 minutes, then wash your face off with warm water. Alternatively, you can turn the potato into a smoothie by blending it. Apply it on your face in a circular motion. Do this raw potato massage at least 3-4 times a week for at least 1 – 2 months, to start seeing remarkable results.

Fenugreek

Fenugreek is anti-inflammatory and is rich in antioxidant and antiseptic properties. The herb is widely used to remedy acne

Get this
- Fenugreek
- Distilled water

Directions
- Mash up the fenugreek leaves and add a little water to make a paste of it. Apply the paste on the acne affected areas and leave it to sit for about 10 to 15 minutes. Wash off your face with warm water afterward. Repeat this process for three to four days to commence healing process.

Indian lilac

Indian lilac contains antiseptic and antimicrobial properties that help kill the bacteria that leads to acne. Lilac also helps soothe the redness and inflammation of skin breakouts. It also serves as a remedy for various skin infections.

Get this
- Turmeric powder
- Indian Lilac
- Water

Directions
- Add turmeric and a little water to powdered lilac to make a paste. Apply the paste on the affected areas. Leave it to sit for about 20 minutes. Rinse off your face with warm water. Alternatively, you can also massage your face with neem oil.

Aspirin Paste

Aspirin paste can be used to exfoliate the skin and kill bacteria causing acne. It contains salicylic acid, an anti-inflammatory agent found in many OTC acne medications.

Get this
- 2 Aspirin Pills
- Water

Directions
- Make a paste of aspirin by crushing it and adding a little water. Apply the paste on your acne/pimples. Leave the mixture on your face for at least 15 minutes. Rinse off with water.

Make a sea salt mixture.

Sea salt helps dry out your pimples and absorb excess oil. It is most effective when mixed with honey

Get this
- One teaspoon of sea salt
- One teaspoon of honey
- Distilled Water

Directions
- Add one teaspoon of sea salt to three three spoons of water. Stir the mixture thoroughly to dissolve the salt. Pour in one teaspoon of honey and stir thoroughly. Gently apply this mixture to your face. Use a Q-tip for application, if you only want it on your pimples. Leave it to sit for about 10minutes. Then rinse off. Apply your moisturizer

Fuller's Earth

Fuller's earth is well known as a cleansing agent. It is widely used to get rid of impurities and dirt particles that clog your skin pores. For centuries, fuller's earth is known to help remedy acne. The clay needed to be mixed with water or rose water and applied on the skin. When used on the skin, fuller earth extracts all hidden dust and dirt particles that clog your pores. It is also a drying agent and helps remove excess oil on the skin.

Get this
- Fuller Earth
- Rose Water
- Sandal Wood Powder

Directions:
- Mix equal proportions of fuller's earth, rose water and sandalwood powder. Apply the mixture on your face. Then wash with warm water. Repeat this process once every week for maximum results

CHAPTER 41

Efficient Remedies to Remove Stretch Marks

The more people find the solutions to their problems, the happier I'm. My goal is to have all the home remedies written in future editions of this book. This chapter covers all treatments for stretch mark. Stretch marks are the pink, red, purple linear streaks that often appear on the abdomen, breast, upper arms, buttocks or thighs.

They usually begin as flat lines and over time they appear as a slightly depressed white streak. Stretch marks can make you feel self-conscious and uncomfortable about your appearance. The appearance is similar to changes seen on an overinflated rubber balloon. They are particularly common among pregnant women, especially during the latter half of pregnancy.

Potato for Stretch Marks:

Potato is believed to help remedy stretch marks. The juice of raw potatoes is said to have a high level of vitamins and minerals, such as vitamin-B complex, Vitamin-C, Calcium, Magnesium, Potassium, Zinc and Phosphorous, that helps speed up the restoration of new skin cells when applied topically. It also contains fatty acids and a wide variety of phytochemicals like carotenoid and polyphenols. Potato juice is also capable of stimulating collagen and elastin synthesis, it can therefore effectively restore skin cells while fading away stretch marks

Materials needed
- 1 medium sized Potato
- Lukewarm water
- Knife

Directions
- Cut the potato into slices. Take the slice and rub it thoroughly over the stretch mark. Leave it to sit for 10 minutes. Then rinse off with lukewarm water

Lemon Juice

Lemon juice is a well-known remedy for improving the appearance of stretch mark. Due to its acidity, it helps remove dead skin cells while developing new cells. Lemon juice also contains enough moisture to help hydrate the skin.

Materials needed
- Lemon
- Warm water
- Cocoa butter
- micro-beads

Directions
- Mix lemon juice with exfoliants such as micro-beads or crushed seed shells and scrub it on the affected area.
- Slice the lemon juice open, squeeze the juice into a bowl and run the lemon juice on the stretch marks in a circular motion. Allow the lemon juice to sit on the skin for about 15 minutes before washing it out.
- Alternatively, you can combine lemon juice with an emollient such cocoa butter. Just place half cup of cocoa butter in a bowl and add 2 tbsp. of lemon juice. Mix thoroughly and apply it to the stretch marks in a circular motion.

- Repeat this therapy for over an extended period, before you can begin to see results

Egg Whites

Egg white is a rich source of amino acids, collagen, and vitamin A, which is very useful for the treatment of scars, burn and stretch marks.

Ways to use Egg White for Stretch Marks
- Whip the white of two eggs gently with a fork. Clean the affected area with warm water and then apply a thick layer of egg white on the stretch mark. Allow the egg white to dry completely on your skin. Then rinse off with warm water. Finally, massage the area with olive oil.

Aloe Vera

Aloe Vera is widely used in many home remedies. The plant has been shown in numerous studies to help heal minor wounds eight days faster than standard dressing. It's also antibacterial and contains vitamins and minerals that can ease eczema and psoriasis flare-ups. Its healing and soothing properties can be used to get rid of stretch marks.

Ways to use Aloe Vera or Stretch Marks
- Remove the outer skin of the aloe vera. Apply the sticky gel on your stretch marks. Let it sit for about two hours. Then wash it off with warm water

Castor Oil

Castor oil is a vegetable oil obtained by pressing the seeds of the castor oil plant. The medicinal and therapeutic benefits of the oil makes it a favorite for home remedies and ayurvedic practices. It contains anti-inflammatory and anti-bacterial properties. It is used as a natural remedy for acne, stretch marks, sunburn, dry skin and also infections like wart, boils, athlete's foot and chronic itching. Castor oil stimulates the production of collagen and elastin. Elastin is a highly elastic protein in connective tissue and allows many tissues in the body to resume their shape after stretching or contracting.

Ways to use Castor Oil
- Apply a generous amount of castor oil to the stretch marks and gently massage the area in a circular motion for at least 5 minutes.
- Apply some heat to the affected area by wrapping the area with a thin cotton cloth, then gently press a hot water bottle or heating pad to it.
- Repeat this process daily for a minimum of one month, to see results

Apricot Mask

Apricot are those beautiful colored fruits full of beta-carotene, vitamins and antioxidant. Apricot can be used as a scrub for rapid removal of stretch marks from the skin.

Ways to use Apricot
- Cut the apricot open and remove the seed from it. Crush the fruit to get their paste. Apply the paste to your stretch marks. Leave to sit for about 15-20 minutes. Wash off with warm water. Repeat this daily for a month

Alfalfa Leaves

Alfalfa leaf contains essential vitamins including the entire spectrum of B-vitamins, A, D, E and K., which helps nourish the skin. Alfalfa Leaf is a source of iron, niacin, biotin, folic acid, calcium, magnesium, phosphorous, potassium, and chlorophyll. It also helps detoxify the urinary tract, purifies the blood and liver.

Ways to use Alfalfa
- Make a paste of alfalfa by crushing it and mixing it up with chamomile oil. Massage the paste into the affected area, two or three times daily. Repeat this daily for a few weeks to see great improvement

Coco-Shea Butter

Coco butter helps nourish your skin and reduce the appearance of stretch marks. It is rich in antioxidants and Vitamin E. The antioxidants and emollient properties of cocoa butter protect skin by limiting the production of free radicals, which can damage skin cells. and also penetrates deep into the skin while repairing it and removing stretch marks. Shear Butter aids coca butter in improving the skin further. Shea butter melts at body temperature, which can be absorbed by the skin fast. Vitamin E in creams is a powerful antioxidant which penetrates through the layers of your skin while assisting natural wound healing process and removing scars.

Materials Needed
- Two tsp Cocoa Butter
- Two tsp Shea Butter
- One tsp Vitamin E oil

Ways to use Shea butter and cocoa butter
- Melt the Shea Butter and Cocoa Butter together
- Pour in the vitamin E to the melted butter

- Mix up thoroughly
- Store in a container (The cream will solidify when left to cool)
- Apply the cream at least twice daily after bath

Alternatively, you can create a blend of cocoa butter, one tablespoon of wheat germ oil, two teaspoons of grated beeswax and one teaspoon of apricot kernel oil and vitamin E oil. Heat the mixture until the beeswax melts. Apply this mixture on your stretch marks two to three times a day. This will hydrate and smoothen your skin

Sugar

Natural white sugar is an excellent source of glycolic acid and alpha hydroxic acid. It stimulates the skin and helps generate younger and fresher looking skin. It can be used to exfoliate the skin and remove dead skin cells. Alpha hydroxic acids are utilized in the treatment of dry skin.
- Mix one tablespoon of raw sugar with one table of lemon juice and almond oil. Apply the mixture to the stretch marks and other skin areas
- Repeat usage after shower each night for at least one month. Your stretch mark will become lighter.

Olive Oil

The various benefits of olive oil are unrivaled, and researchers reveal more and more benefits every day. Olive oil is rich in vitamin A, and E. Vitamin E helps to neutralize the oxidant effect of free radicals that damage collagen, which is the primary reason for stretch marks. While Vitamin A thickens and stimulates the dermis and reduces stretch marks by increasing blood flow to the surface of the skin. Olive oil is also widely used as a solution to stretch mark during pregnancy. By massaging the area with luke warm olive oil, helps speed up the blood circulation over the area. Leave the oil on the skin for at least one hour so that the skin can absorb the vitamin of the oil properly. The idea here is that your skin will soften, and when it softens, it expands, and, in general, goes with the punches more easily. This remedy should be followed by at least one month, for an effective difference.

Water

Keeping your body hydrated always helps protect your body from several kinds of illness and also aids in detoxification and restoring skin elasticity. To keep the body hydrated, drink at least 8 to 10 glasses of water per day. Drinking water regularly can help stretch mark fade but may not completely remove it.

CHAPTER 42

Removing blackhead with home remedies.

I can still recall am an incident that took place at a supermarket sometime in 2013. I was standing beside a particular lady, who was about to pay a huge sum for a blackhead cream. I couldn't help but tell her that I have a better alternative for blackhead, but she immediately passed it off saying, "I can't be caught dead apply such on my face" At that moment I felt undermined. Gradually, I left her sight.

Most of us are still making the same mistake. We have so much confidence these chemical formulated creams, and we refuse to see that they are the leading cause of our problems.

Blackhead is caused by hair follicles that get clogged with oil, dead skin cells, and other impurities. As there is not much skin to attach to, they become open to air. The top layer then oxidizes and turn a dark black color. Below is the list of my fantastic blackhead remedy.

The Honey Remedy

Cleopatra was well known for her flawless skin. Her major secret was honey. Honey pulls away dirt from skin pores while nourishing and moisturizing the skin to maintain it's shine. Its antioxidant, antiseptic and antibacterial properties make it the best alternative to removing blackhead. Warm a generous amount of honey and apply it on the affected area. Leave it on your skin for about 10 to 15 minutes. Wash off afterward. The natural cleansing property of honey will clear the blackheads and

Honey and Milk Pore Strips

I read somewhere on the web that Cleopatra used this remedy to maintain a flawless skin. History made us believe that she bathed with milk and honey. These two ingredients are very common in every facial treatment. Milk is rich in lactic acid which is said to help keep skin soft and supple.

You will need.
- One teaspoon of milk
- One tablespoon of raw organic honey
- Clean strip of cotton

Directions:
Heat the mixture of the specified portion of honey and milk for about 5-10 seconds in your microwave. Mix thoroughly again and leave to cool. Gently apply a thin layer over blackhead and pat a strip of clean, dry cotton on it. Leave it to dry for about 25 minutes and carefully peel the strip away. Rinse your face with water and moisturize with coconut oil (optional)

Egg White Mask

My mom's favorite remedy for removing blackheads. Egg white helps tighten your pores and remove dirt that has clogged up over time. Egg white is rich in protein and provides the skin with the needed nutrients.

You will need
- 1 egg
- Toilet paper
- A small bowl
- A clean towel

Directions:
Carefully beat your egg open and be careful not to mix up the white with the yolk. With your fingertips gently apply the egg white on the affected areas. Then, take two plies of toilet paper and place on it, while using your fingers to press down on it. Leave it on till the paper becomes stiff. Then apply a second layer of egg white over the tissue, let it dry. You can also apply a third layer, which is entirely optional. Now, gently pull off the tissue and wash your face to remove residues.

Baking Soda

Baking soda is highly efficient in the treatment of black head. It's mild abrasive helps in cleaning the skin and removing blackheads. Baking soda helps to neutralize the skin's pH level while reducing the excess oil produced by the skin. Baking soda can also be used to exfoliate the skin, leaving it soft and supple.

You need:
- Baking Soda
- Water
- Apple Cider Vinegar

Directions:
Start by washing your face with warm water to open up the skin pores. Then make a thick paste of baking soda by mixing it with few drops of water. Apply the paste to your face, with more attention on the affected area. Let it sit for a few minutes. Then massage it thoroughly on the face -in a circular motion. Doing this helps loosen the dead skin cells. Rinse off with warm water. Repeat this twice a week for best results. Another great alternative is the baking soda and vinegar.

Mix apple cider vinegar with baking soda to form a paste. Apply this mixture to your face by spreading a thick layer using your fingertips. Make sure to avoid the areas under eyes. Let it dry off; this usually takes up to 20 minutes. Make sure to keep your head up to prevent dry chunks from falling off your face. You may begin to experience some itchy sensation, don't panic, the mask is soaking up the facial impurities and pulling it away from your skin. Then rinse your face with warm water and wash off with your cleanser of choice, then moisturize.

Sugar Scrub:

Most of the time all you need is to exfoliate your skin, followed by adding your moisturizer of choice. Exfoliating the skin helps get rid of dead skin cells that clog up your pores, thereby leading to blackheads. You mustn't break your bank to get the ingredients ready, all that is needed are simple ingredients

Sugar Scrub Ingredients
- 1/2 cup sugar, white or brown sugar
- 1/2 cup oil, Olive oil or coconut oil can work

Directions
Mix all ingredients and store in an airtight jar. You can now scrub your skin with the mixture and rinse will. It will leave your skin feeling like silk.

Lemon

Lemon is another excellent remedy for blackhead. Lemon is rich in alpha-hydroxy acid which naturally prevents acne, blackheads, pimples and other skin problems. It is very effective in removing excess oil from the skin while nourishing and brightening the skin complexion. Its acidic properties help exfoliate and cleanse oily skin, preventing bacterial and other infections.

You need:
- Lemon juice
- Cotton ball
- Water
- Baking soda (Second Alternative)
- Brown sugar (Second Alternative)

Directions:
Extract the juice of a lemon in a small bowl and dilute with a small amount of water. Apply juice directly to skin with the aid of a cotton ball. Allow it to dry up naturally, then wash off. Repeat this process 2-3 times daily for best results.
Alternative, use lemon, baking soda, and baking soda. Baking soda exfoliates and removes dead skin cells and blackheads from the skin. To do this mix baking soda and granulated brown sugar in a bowl and add freshly squeezed lemon juice. Stir the mixture properly until thoroughly blended. Apply to damp skin and gently scrub and massage with your fingers. After the scrubbing let it sit for about 10 -15 minutes. Then rinse with lukewarm water. Do this twice weekly for best results

Steam It Out

Steaming helps reduce the appearance of blackhead by softening up trapped sebum/dead skin cells that fill out your pores and form blackhead.

You need:
- Water
- A clean, soft towel
- A large bowl

Directions:
Start by filling your bowl with boiling water. Let it cool a little bit, cover your head with a large towel and lean towards the bowl of hot water, forming a tent-like shape. Don't get too close to the hot water to avoid burning your face. After which you rinse your face with warm water and pat dry. Then moisturize

CHAPTER 43

Amazing treatment for Uterine Fibroid

Uterine Fibroid is a non-cancerous tumor that forms within the walls of a woman's uterus. They usually form in various sizes; some can be as tiny as a full stop while some can get as large as the size of a grapefruit.

Most women with fibroid never get to know they have one. Some get to discover the presence of fibroid during their routine pelvic examination. In most cases fibroid tumors cause no symptoms. But with some women, they experience heavy menstrual bleeding, bleeding between period, constant pain the abdomen, frequent urination, increased virginal discharge, lower back pain, and pain during sexual intercourse.

Fibroid does not interrupt the menstrual cycle, but they can cause infertility or miscarriage. Fibroid tends to form during a woman's late thirties and early forties and shrinks after menopause. Please do note that fibroid is not in any way associated with cancer and those not increase the woman's risk of uterine cancer; so banish the fear of any linkage to cancer. Fibroid is a natural occurrence in every woman, and it's estimated that 20 to 50 percent of women of reproductive age have fibroids. The fluctuation in levels of estrogen and progesterone which are the two primary female sex hormone influences fibroid growth. However while all women produce estrogen, only some do develop the fibroid tumors. Fibroid is most common among African women. The causes of fibroid are still unknown, but some factors can influence the growth of fibroid.

Hormones: Estrogen and progesterone are the hormones produced by the ovaries. They cause the uterine lining to regenerate during each menstrual cycle and may stimulate the growth of fibroids.

Family History: Sometimes fibroid may be genetic. If your mother, sister, or grandmother has a history of this condition, you may develop it as well.

Pregnancy: Pregnancy increases the production of estrogen and progesterone in your body. Fibroids may develop and grow rapidly while you are pregnant.

Small fibroids do not necessary need any cause for panic or treatments. The big ones are the major problem, which requires treatment from a physician or the application of natural remedies. Their positions within the uterus determine their names.

- Intrauterine fibroids are located within the uterus
- Submucosal fibroids are located in the walls of the uterus.
- Subserosal fibroids are located under the serous membrane of the uterus.

• Alternative Treatments to fibroid

Green Tea

Green tea extract (epigallocatechin gallate) has being shown in clinical trials to reduce the severity of fibroids symptoms. Women who take green tea will experience fewer severe symptoms and fibroid size shrank by over 30%.

- Take 240 mg 3 times daily, or decaffeinated tea bag prepared with 1 cup of water.
- Take 1 cup 2-3 times daily. To avoid dilution, please do not use within an hour of taking other medications.

Please note that the caffeine in green tea might cause insomnia, anxiety, upset stomach, nausea or diarrhea.

Flaxseed:

Flaxseed contains plant based hormones called phytoestrogen which is a safer alternative to synthetic hormones and decreases the effect of estrogen levels naturally by blocking the estrogen receptors on the cells in fibroid and other estrogen-sensitive tissues. Also studies have shown that eating flaxseed helps the body reduce the production of unhealthy estrogens. The omega-3 fatty acid and fiber found in flaxseed help reduce inflammations and tumor growth throughout the body, ridding the body of excess estrogen.

Herbs:

Vitex (Vitex Agnus-Castus)

Vitex promotes the production of progesterone by reducing estrogen levels. For best results, take vitex for at least three months

To make vitex tea: Pour three cups of boiling water over two tablespoons of crushed vitex berries. Steep for 20 minutes, strain, and drink three cups a day.
Vitex has a spicy, and peppery taste. You can also take one-half teaspoon of liquid extract or two capsules, three times daily.

Dandelion Root (Taraxacum Officinale)

Dandelion root affects the liver by improving bile flow, which in turns leads to efficient degradation of excess estrogen, flushed out of the body. For best results, take dandelion for at least three months.
To make Dandelion root tea: Simmer three tablespoons of dandelion root in three cups of water for 15 minutes in a covered pot. Remove from heat and let stand for an additional 15 minutes. Strain, and drink three cups a day.
Dandelion root has an earthy, slightly bitter flavor. You can also take 1 to 2 teaspoons of liquid extract or two capsules three times daily.

Milk thistle (Silybum Marianum)

Milk thistle works on the liver by promoting the regeneration of liver cells. Which helps to maintain active liver function.
For best results, take an extract of milk thistle, standardized for silymarin, which is considered to be the primary active ingredient.

Take 140 milligrams of silymarin three times daily for at least three months. If you prefer to use the whole herb, you can grind milk thistle seeds in a coffee grinder and sprinkle them on cereals, salads, or other dishes. Eat approximately two tablespoons daily.

Nettle (Urtica Dioica)

It contains iron and other natural elements, which promotes the production of new red blood cells thus counteracting anemia caused by excessive bleeding. Nettle is safe and gentle and can be taken indefinitely.

To make nettle tea: Pour 3 cups of boiling water over two tablespoons of dried nettle, cover, and steep for 15 minutes. Strain, and drink three cups daily.

Yellow Dock (Rumex Crispus)

Yellow dock is an amazing purifying herb. It improves liver function by stimulating bile flow and has mild laxative properties. It acts as a tonic which promotes the production of blood cells thus correcting anemia caused by excessive bleeding.

To make yellow dock tea: Simmer 2 tablespoons of dried root in 3.5 cups of water for 15 minutes in a covered pot. Remove from heat and steep for an additional 10 minutes. Strain and sweeten (if desired), and drink 3 cups daily.

Yellow dock has a bitter, earthy flavor. If you prefer, you can take 0.5 teaspoon of liquid extract or 2 capsules three times a day.

Red Raspberry

Red Raspberry is used in controlling irregular menstrual bleeding while strengthening the uterine muscles. Red Raspberry is useful in helping the body return balance to the reproductive organs. Also, it offers anti-inflammatory and anti-emetic effects making Red Raspberry a powerful herb for easing menstrual symptoms related to uterine fibroids. It is a rich source of nutrients which includes calcium, magnesium, iron, potassium, phosphorus, and vitamins A, B, C and E. This is a very useful tonic for women suffering from severe menstrual symptoms.

Herbal Tea (Red Clover)

Herbal teas suggested for the treatment of uterine fibroids include a tea brewed from the blooms of the red clover herb. Red clover is rich in phytoestrogens. Red Clover inhibits the growth of uterine tissue making it an effective way to treat the uterine fibroids. Drink 2 to 3 cups of red clover tea to help shrink uterine fibroids.

Other Herbs you should know

Black cohosh: Tablets, take 250-500 mg daily, to stop bleeding and relieves pain, especially leg pain

Cinnamon: Oil, 5 – 10 drops every 15 minutes for up to 4 hours or until bleeding subsides, to reduce fibroid bleeding.

Dan Shen: use this under the supervisor of a professional. It helps treat congealed blood and pelvic congestion.

Reishi: Tincture: Take 1 tbsp (12 ml) in ¼ cup water three times daily to stop pelvic inflammation. Useful if there is emotional tension
Red Clover and Burdock root: Both helps in the cleansing of the bloodstream

Herbal Treatment Alternative for Uterine Fibroids:

Herbal Bath

This is an alternative topical method to treat uterine fibroids. For practical use prepare a warm sitz bath. Pour in 1 to 2 cups of herbal tea decoction brewed from Mexican wild yams into the water. Sit in the bath for 10 to 15 minutes; repeat twice a day. Herbal tea infusion brewed from horsetail can be substituted for Mexican wild yam.

Essential Oil Supplements

Herbal essential oil like evening primrose oil is rich in omega 6 fatty acids, powerful antioxidants, and anti-inflammatory substances. Primrose oil can help reduce pain and inflammation of fibroids. Evening primrose essential oil is available in supplemental form at health food stores.

Avoid High estrogen foods:

The estrogen hormone feeds the fibroid; that's why it vanished with menopause. Most commercially sold food like red meat, poultry, dairy products, eggs contains synthetic estrogen, feed to them routinely for market purposes. These estrogen rich foods should be avoided throughout your healing period and organic hormone free dairy, egg and meat should be used instead.

Decrease the intake of white food:

Food such as white bread and pasta increases insulin, thereby changing the way estrogen is metabolized. They create compounds that are more likely to cause cellular inflammation and fibroid symptoms, including enhanced growth of existing fibroid.

Consume more fiber and soy:

Fiber helps the liver process and excrete excess estrogen. Therefore, high fiber foods like grains, beans, vegetable, and fruits should regularly be consumed. Also, I recommend you concentrate on soybeans products like soymilk, tofu, and soy sauce. Soy is rich in natural estrogen called phytoestrogens, a compound that is 100 times weaker than synthetic estrogen, so they do no harm to the body, but instead binds to estrogen receptor sites while preventing harmful synthetic estrogen from damaging your system.

Acupuncture:

This practice can be used to shrink fibroid tumor substantially. Stimulating the proper acupuncture point can help shrink fibroid.

Chinese Medicine:

Chinese medicine has been shown substantially to shrink the size of the fibroid tumor and reduce symptoms. Well-known Chinese herbal remedy Kuei-chin-fu-ling-wan was shown to reduce fibroid size in about 60%. Several other studies have shown that Tripterygium wilfordii extract or lei gong teng, can shrink fibroids better than the drug mifepristone.

Caution:

If your menstrual bleeding is so heavy and saturates your sanitary pad more often than an hour, please consult a health practitioner.

If fibroid is found, please do not take oral contraceptives with high estrogen content. Because high estrogen birth control may stimulate the growth of fibroid tumors.

CHAPTER 44

Colon Cleansing Made Easy

I have numerous experiences with different kinds of detox cleanse. Sometime in the past, that should be the 2013 Christmas holidays; I went to spend the holidays with my family and my toxic colon ruined the whole moment for me. The annoying part was that it choose the wrong time to strike. Exactly on Christmas Eve, I felt a severe headache, low energy, constipated, fatigue and low energy level.

This event made me miss out on the Christmas turkey and other goodies my mom prepared. On the 25th day, a day after Christmas, I still felt the same way. It was evident it's time to see a doctor, so I went to the family physician. After many check-ups, he gave me a list of Pills to take. I heeded to his advice, even though I never believed they work. Although I had an instant relieve with them. As soon as I stopped, it all came back again, even worse than before. I knew for once that there must be an alternative remedy for my case, but the question was which remedy? All I needed was to connect the symptoms to a particular treatment. After much ado, I found out that the cause of my problem was toxins in my colon. Toxins from your gastrointestinal tract can lead to a variety of health problems such as allergies, asthma, and arthritis. With proper colon cleansing comes with improved health, high energy level, and healthy immune system.

3 Days Apple Juice Fast

If doing an Enema is too much of a big deal for you, another alternative is a one or three days apple juice fast. Apple juice happens to be one the best remedy to cleanse your colon, it encourages bowel movement and breaks down toxins. I strongly recommend apple juice fast, because your digestive system will be put to rest while allowing for thorough detoxification of your colon. If apple juice is too boring for you, feel free to spice is up with lemon or any vegetable of your choice. Regular intake of water while on the fast is recommended. Personal, I have a habit of taking at least 3 cups of water first thing every morning upon waking up; after which I have my breakfast an hour later; doing this hold immense health benefits. I owe my glowing skin to that. You can also pick up that habit at zero cost. Another thing you should also consider during your fast is the lemon infused water which I wrote about in the previous chapter. Infused water holds immense detoxification benefits too; if you have made up your mind to include it, do it first thing in the morning, upon waking up. If you are not ok with a juice fast idea, you can go on a smoothie fast, this time, you use a blender, not a juicer. You can also mix up with an apple diet (sliced, peeled, whole, chilled or normal) and virgin coconut oil (My favorite of them all). After the fast, don't rush into solid meals, just go on salads on the fourth day and gradually introduce solid meals. Rushing into solid food can give you severe stomach upset, for a longer fast, it can land you in the hospital.

Sea Salt

The salt water flush is most effective if you perform it first thing in the morning on an empty stomach. If you do it later in the day, just make sure you haven't eaten anything in the past one to two hours. Ideally, perform the flush before you eat breakfast, but be careful if you plan to leave the house or exercise in the morning — you'll have a strong desire to go to the bathroom shortly after and might have a queasy stomach after the flush.
Sea salt is not one of my favorite colon cleansing remedies, but it's worth the try. Most naturopathic doctors believe that it's one of the most efficient colon cleansing remedies. But experts recommends that you do it on an empty stomach. Please also

do not that there are some precautions around this remedy. If you are a patient of high blood pressure or have any heart-related disease, I suggest you abstain from this remedy. If you must, consult your physician first. Also taking too much of it can cause diarrhea. Sea salt stimulates the bowel movement while removing all harmful toxin that gets accumulated in fecal matter.

Direction:

Bring a glass of water to boil (just place the glass of water in a pot of boiling water), then add one tablespoon of sea salt, and let it boil some more. Bring it out from heat and let it cool to a degree you can easily sip. Gradually sip the solution. You may feel mild nausea or a headache. Then gently massage your stomach. After some time you will begin to feel the need to visit the toilet, it only shows that the toxins in your colon are ready to get away. It's now time to lay on your bed and rest. If you plan on embarking on this remedy, I suggest you take the day off, because you will need a lot of rest. After the needed rest fill up your system to make up for the lost minerals, water and electrolyte due to the salt water. I glass of green juice, or smoothie wouldn't hurt!

Triphala (Ayurvedic Herbal Remedy for Colon Cleansing)

Triphala is yet another very useful herb for colon cleansing widely used in Ayurvedic practise. It is a combination of two terms, Phala which means fruits and Tri meaning three. I have not tried this remedy before, but those that have can testify it works. Triphala helps promote bowel movement, which leads to the elimination toxic waste in the body, it does this due to the presence of Bioflavonoids, Vitamin C, Linoleic oil and phospholipids.

Directions:

Add a tablespoon of Triphala into a glass of water and drink the solution every morning, at least for three days. If you are still wondering where to get this herb, it can be found in Ayurveda health stores or online Ayurveda shops.

Water

I can overemphasize the usefulness of water to the body. We live in a world where we only drink water when we are dehydrated. Water goes a long way to help your muscle cells perform well and help keep your skin looking good. It also does and fantastic job of aiding your kidney cleanse and rid your body of toxins. When you hydrate yourself properly thing moves fine through your gastrointestinal tract and prevent constipation. When you don't, the colon pulls water from your stool to maintain hydration, which may result in constipation. Of late I have been doing my water therapy and two weeks in it, I observed few unusual changes ranging from a glowing skin to a good bowel movement.

Fruits and Vegetables high in fiber- for everyday colon cleansing

If you are the type that gets your adequate serving of fruits and vegetable, you don't have much worry about colon cleansing. The fiber in these fruits and vegetables automatically does the job for you. Fibers in vegetables and fruits encourage your body to expel waste products while keeping your colon clean.

Lemon Juice

Lemon juice is another remedy worth giving a try; it contains a powerhouse of antioxidant and Vitamin C, which is excellent for your digestive system. Add a pinch of salt and honey into a glass of lemon juice. Pour lukewarm water into the glass and stir it properly. Drink this mixture on an empty stomach, ever morning. You can also add apple juice to the mix and drink three times daily; This will help thin out the mucus in your bowel.

CHAPTER 45

Reversing Diabetes

It was indeed a sad day for everybody, as we sat in the hospital waiting for the dreadful act about to be done to Uncle John to save his life. I couldn't believe this was happening to him. Uncle John is a very nice guy.

Growing up, I still remember how Uncle John never missed giving gifts to my siblings and me. I couldn't hold back my tears watching Aunty Theresa Uncle John's wife on the floor in a pool of her tears. Uncle John was about to get his lower limbs amputated because his type II diabetics had just gotten worse. The doctor said that the nerves in Uncle Sam's feet was damaged and had become numb due to the high glucose levels that had accumulated over time resulting in a condition called diabetic neuropathy. Before this, Uncle John had developed blisters and small wounds on his foot. We thought it was something we could dress with hydrogen peroxide and leave nature to take its course, but over time, we observed that things were getting worse. We decided to pull the red flag and take Uncle John to the hospital. That's when we got the dreadful news of amputation. Before then, I used to think diabetics was a joke. I never knew it could result in something as severe as amputation. Diabetes, when left untreated, can also lead to other diseases, such as kidney disease, blood vessel damage, infections, heart disease, nerve damage, high blood pressure, blindness, and even strokes. That was just my encounter with type 2 diabetics. Let me also narrate my encounter with type 1 diabetics. Type 1 diabetics is when your body stops producing insulin, the hormone that helps your body cells utilize blood sugar. Mrs. Edwin is a good friend of my mom. Her 1-year-old son was diagnosed with type 1 diabetics, and the poor boy is now going to live insulin dependent for the rest of his life. How did this come about? Mrs. Edwin is a busy executive with a Fortune 500 company and thought she was too busy to cater for her baby, so she left him in the care of her maid, who fed the baby with nothing but cow's milk. I think it's wise that if your family has any history type 1 diabetics, keep cow's milk as far away as possible from your children. Type 1 diabetics is not only hereditary but can be encouraged in infants by feeding them with cow's milk. According to a study by Johana Paronen from Helsinki Finland on children diagnosed with type 1 diabetics. It states that type 1 diabetics on infants, may not be an autoimmune disease, but an intense allergic reaction to cow's milk and the antibodies created during that allergic reaction also cross-react with islet cells of the pancreas, therefore destroying them. Type 1 diabetics can also be caused in an infant by a mother who had pre-eclampsia (a condition characterized by a sharp increase in blood pressure during the third trimester of pregnancy) or viral infections during infancy, including mumps, rubella, and coxsackie.

People living with diabetes are also advised to keep away from gluten. An animal-based study conducted at the Mayo Clinic proposed that eating gluten can increase your risk of diabetes. Gluten triggers a hereditary allergic condition called celiac disease, a severe intestinal illness associated with the development of type 2 diabetes. It best to fill your plate with lean meats, fruits, and vegetables that reduce inflammation and keep you healthy.

*****Type 1 diabetes can be managed, but not sure if it can be cured. But with type 2 diabetes, there are several claims that it can be reversed through home remedies. Personal I have seen a man who managed type 2 diabetes for over 30 years without medications and he is in strong health. He owes this to his routine exercise and healthy eating habits. Individuals who are physically inactive or overweight are much more likely to develop type 2 diabetes.

Fenugreek Remedies for Diabetes

Fenugreek is one herb I know for sure that helps lowering blood sugar level. Indians widely use it and it's mostly grown in South Asia, North Africa and parts of the Mediterranean. Several type 2 diabetics clinical trials conducted on Fenugreek has shown that it can reduce the rate at which sugar is absorbed during digestion. It also helps in insulin production by stimulating the cells in the pancreas gland. Fenugreek owes its power to an amino acid called 4-hydroxyisoleucine. This amino acid has been extracted and purified from fenugreek seeds, which are known in traditional medicine for their antidiabetic properties. 4-Hydroxyisoleucine increases glucose-induced insulin release, in the concentration range of 100 micromol/l to 1 mmol/l, through a direct effect on isolated islets of Langerhans from both rats and humans.

How to use Fenugreek for Diabetes

- Start by roasting fenugreek seed. Placing them in a large skillet and heating on medium heat for about two minutes (Stir Frequently) Then, add two table-spoons of the roasted seeds to Indian curries and Asian stir-fry dishes.

- You can as well steep two tablespoons of dried fenugreek leaves and seed in 1 cup of boiling water and leave for 10 minutes. Strain the liquid and drink the resulting mixture twice per day.

- Another way is to pour water over four tablespoons of dried fenugreek seed and leaves. Let it steep for about 30 minutes, to produce a tincture. You can take half of the tincture three times per day.

- Two tablespoons of fenugreek seeds powder can be added to a glass of milk or warm water. Drink this every day

- Another effective way to take Fenugreek is to mix six tablespoons of fenugreek to three tablespoons of turmeric powder. Soak the mixture in water overnight. Sieve out the resulting liquid and drink

Bilberry Extract

Bilberry's are dark blue fruits that look more like blueberries, but a bit smaller and softer. Both the leaves and ripe fruit are using in the treatment of type II diabetics. The leaves are well known to help control blood sugar. They do this by impairing the normal process in the liver. Because of this, I wouldn't suggest the use of the leaves for a long term treatment. The berries help lower blood sugar and take it even further by improving the strength and integrity of the blood vessels while reducing the damage to these vessels associated with diabetes and other diseases such as atherosclerosis.

Bitter Gourd

Bitter Gourd is a tropical and subtropical vine of the family of Cucurbitaceae, widely grown in Asia and Africa. It has many varieties, and it's extremely bitter. Bitter Gourd is one of the most efficient remedies for diabetes and widely used in Asian countries. Many types of research have been conducted on Bitter ground which proved its effectiveness on blood sugar level, enhancing the sensitivity of insulin and encourages the glucose metabolism to all over the body. Thus increasing the pancreatic insulin secretion and preventing insulin resistance. Bitter gourd is rich in plant insulin – polypeptide, which has a biochemical that is very useful in reducing the blood sugar. It

Ways to have Bitter Melon or Bitter Gourd for Diabetes
- Peel and remove the seeds of 5 bitter gourds. Place them in a juicer and juice out the liquid content. If you don't have a juicer, you can use a blender. But remember to seize out the liquid content with a mesh strainer when using a blender. Drink the fresh juice on an empty stomach, every morning

- Cook bitter gourd in ghee and take it frequently. To do this start by cutting the bitter melon into pieces. Then add ghee or clarified butter to a cooking pan and pour bitter gourd into the pan. Place the pan on heat and cook for a few minutes. Do this for about four months for complete relief of diabetes.

- You can also add one tablespoon of amla juice to one cup of bitter gourd juice and take this portion for few months.

Cinnamon Remedies for Diabetes

A 2012 study conducted reveals that cinnamon had a potentially beneficial effect on glycemic control. While another study published in 2009, found that a 500 mg capsule of cinnamon taken twice daily for 90 days improved hemoglobin A1C levels. Which is a reflection of average blood sugar level for the past two to three months in people with poorly controlled type 2. Also, since diabetics are naturally prone to cardiovascular diseases, it makes total sense that taking cinnamon has can help lower the risk of cardio diseases. Cinnamon powder lowers blood sugar by stimulating insulin activity. Please note that the best type of cinnamon to go for is the Ceylon cinnamon which is a safer alternative than it's cheaper counterpart, Cassia cinnamon. Cassia cinnamon contains a compound called coumarin. Coumarin is toxic and can cause damage to your liver and its functioning.

Ways to use Cinnamon Powder for Diabetes
- Pour water into a pan and place the pan on heat. Then add the cinnamon stick to the water and allow it to boil for a few minutes before turning off the flame. Let it steep for about 20 minutes. Strain the water and drink it. Do this daily till you begin to see improvement

- You can also add one tablespoon of cinnamon powder in 1 cup of warm water. Drink this daily.

- Cinnamon powder can also be sprinkled on your salads, dips or other dishes.

Aloe Vera Remedy for Diabetes

I have known about this Aleo Vera treatment since I was a kid. I helped my grandmother grow a lot of them in her backyard. Most of the time she will instruct me to take some to patients at their homes. Modern researcher has found that Aloe vera is highly beneficial in lowering blood glucose and blood lipid levels in diabetics patients. Also helps in reducing fasting blood sugar levels. Its hypoglycemic activity has proven to be highly useful in both insulin-dependent diabetes and non-insulin dependent diabetes.

Ways to use Aloe Vera for Diabetes

- For this method, you will need one tablespoon of Aloe Vera gel, one tablespoon of Bay Leaves Powder and one tablespoon of Tumeric powder. When all these ingredients are complete, add the bay leaves powder and turmeric powder into the aloe vera gel. Mix thoroughly. Drink this mixture daily

- Another way is to add buttermilk to freshly squeezed aloe vera and stir well, till it forms a thick consistency. Drinking daily to help with diabetics

Lady Finger for Diabetes

Lady finger is also known as okra and used in preparing soup in Nigeria. It is high in vitamin A, B6, C, K, Magnesium, Potassium, Zinc and soluble fiber. You might be wondering what makes okra so potent for Diabetes. Its fiber content helps in regulating the rate at which sugar is absorbed from your intestinal tract while the seed is rich in alpha-glucosidase inhibitors. Alpha-glucosidase inhibitors stop starch from converting into glucose.

How to use lady finger for diabetes?

- You will need two to three okra pods and one glass of water. Start by washing your okra pods. Cut off the head and tail of your okra pods. Then split it open vertically from the middle and immerse both ends in a glass filled with water. Cover and let it soak overnight. Early in the morning drink the water on an empty stomach. Do this daily for a couple of months; you will see dramatic improvement

Papaya Leaf Remedies for Diabetes

It will amaze you to know that papaya is another excellent remedy for diabetes. It does this by increasing insulin sensitivity; this reduces the enzyme levels of ATL and AST, which are the bio makers of type – 2 diabetes for improving insulin sensitivity so that cells can effectivity take glucose. The antioxidant found in papaya leaf extract helps in decreasing the secondary complications of diabetes such as fatty liver, kidney damage and oxidative stress. Also consuming papaya leaves improves the process of wound healing in diabetic due to its anti-bacterial and antioxidant action

How to use Papaya Leaf for Diabetics
Start by getting all your ingredients ready.
- Ten leaves of Papaya
- Eight cups of water.

Directions:
- Put the papaya leaves into the water and boil the water till it is half of its quantity.
- Leave it to cool for a while.
- Drink this concoction in small doses throughout the day. You will get some added benefits by drinking this tea. It helps cure indigestion and boost immune system

Mango Leaves Remedies for Diabetes

Before now you believe that mango leaves are not edible. But to your surprise, they are. In Nigeria, some herbalist use mango leaves in the treatment of diabetes. Its aqueous extract has hypoglycemic activity which lowers the intestinal absorption of glucose, therefore improves blood lipid profiles. To get the maximum benefits from mango leaves, it's recommended that you consume it 60 minutes before eating.

How to use Mango Leaves for Diabetes

Simply soak 15 mango leaves in a glass of water and leave it overnight. Upon waking up in the morning drink the resulting solution on an empty stomach and have your breakfast one hour later. Alternatively, place few mango leave under the sun to get it dried up. When it is completely dried, grind them to a powdered form and store in a container and have ½ of this powered leaves daily before launch.

Get Physical

If you have diabetics, exercising is your best bet to manage diabetics, maintain optimum health, and control blood sugar level. Exercise will help you lose weight and reverse your symptoms of type 2 diabetics. You mustn't start with heavy weights, just having a short walk early in the morning can go a long way.

Change your Diet

Even if you use all the home remedies above and still do not maintain a healthy diet, all efforts will be in vain. To adequately manage type 2 diabetics and live a healthful life, you need to avoid certain foods. Food rich in refined floor should be replaced with whole wheat bread and whole wheat pasta. Eat brown rice in place of polished rice. Use low-fat dairy products, like skimmed milk, cheese, and yogurt. Ginger is also good for reversing type 2 diabetics, and it's advised you take ½ tsp of ginger juice and ½ tsp garlic juice, mixed with a little honey or jaggery, twice a day. Include garlic, onion, bitter gourd, spinach, raw banana, black plum in your diet. Food with high carbohydrates, like potatoes, sweet potatoes, yam, oily and spicy foods.

Index

A

Air freshener 47
alismol. *See* magnim
alkaline 35
aloe vera gel 40
antacids 40
antibacterial 38
anti-inflammatory 44
apple cider vinegar 39

B

baking soda 34
   Improves Skin Complexion 37
   itching and burning 37
    sodium bicarbonate 35
   Teeth Whitener 36
   Treats Sunburn 37
Benefits of Enemas 50
bicarbonate 38
bile 51
blood pressure 40
Body Odour 38
Boiling Chicken 48

C

caffeinated beans 51
candida albicans 40
Canker Sore 44
Carpet Deodorizer 45
choleretics 51
Cleaning Agent 46
Clean Kitchen Utensils 47
coconut oil 37
colon 39, 50

D

Dandruff 38
dead skin cells 37
Deodorize Garbage Cans 48
Diaper Rash 41
discharge 40
Dr. Max Gerson 51
Dry Shampoo 45

E

enema bag 51
Erase Crayon 48
euissenim. *See* lamet
exfoliating agent 37
Exfoliator 42

F

Facial Scrub 46
faeces. 51
Fast oxidizers 51
fecal matters 50
feuguer. *See* television
Freshen Sponges 45
fungus 40

G

glutathione 51
grandmother's journal 35

H

hairbrush 46
Hand Cleanser 42
Heartburn 41
house cleansers 35
hydrogen peroxide 39

I
Improves Skin Complexion 37
Indigestion 41
Insect Bites 41

J
juicing enthusiast 48

K
Keep Ants Out 48
Keep Flowers Fresher Longer 49
kitchen scrub 44

L
lactic acid 42
large intestine 51
lavender oil 46
lemon juice. 40
liver 51

M
magnim. *See* adiam
microorganism 40
mild antiseptic 37
Modelling Clay 47
mouth sores 44

N
Nail Cleaner 46
Natural Oven Cleaning 47
Neutralize Gassy Beans 48
neutralizes stomach acid 37

O
oily scalp 38

P
Pamper Your Feet 44
Pedicure 46
peristalsis 50
Poison Ivy 41
Produce Wash 48

Q
queasy stomach 40

R
Relaxing Soak 42
Remove Blackheads 43
Remove Chlorine from Hair 46

S
sequis. *See* sendipissi
Silver Polish 47
skin irritation 41
slow oxidizers 51
Smelly Shoes 46
Soften Fabric 47
Splinter Remover 42

T
Teeth Whitener 36
Toilet Odour 45
Tomatoes 43
toxic waste 51
toxins 51
Treats Sunburn 37
turmeric root powder 36

U
Ulcer 37
unclogging pores 43

Upset Stomach 40
utat. *See* nulputpat

V
vagina 40
Volumizing Shampoo 45
vulva 40

Y
yatiscili. *See* praesse
Yeast Infection 40
Yellow Nails 39
yuiscili. *See* odio

Bibliography

Encyclopedia of Natural Medicine. Michael Murray, N.D and Joseph Pizzomo, N.D. Rocklin, CA: Prima Publishing, 1991.

Prescription for Nutritional Healing. Phyllis A. Balch, CNC: Published by Penguin Group, 1930-2004

The Juicing bible. Pat Croker: Published by Robert Rose Inc, 2000, 2008

Prescription for Herbal Healing. Phyllis A. Balch, CNC: Published by Penguin Group, 2012

Alternative Cures. Bill Gottlieb: The Random House Publishing, 2000

The Gerson Therapy: The Amazing Juicing Programme for Cancer and other illness

The Complete Book of Juicing: Michael Murray N.D: Clark Potter/Publishers New York, 2013

Sodium Bicarbonate: Nature's Unique First Aid Remedy. Mark Sircus: Square One Publishers, 2014

Healing Psoriasis: The Natural Alternative. John O. A. Pagano: Published by John Wiley & Sons, 2009.

The Healing Powers of Honey: Cal Orey: Published by Kensington Publishing Corporation.

The Healing Powers of Vinegar: A Complete Guide To Nature's most remarkable remedy, revised and updated. Published by Kensington Publishing Corp. 2000, 2006

Aloe Vera Handbook: The Acient Egyptian Medicine Plant: Max B. Skousen

The Coconut Oil Miracle, 5th Edition. By Bruce Fife, C.N., N.D

Turmeric and the Healing Curcuminoids. By Muhammed Majeed, 1996

The Natural Remedies Encyclopedia. By M.D. Vance H. Ferrell and Harold M. Cherne

Prescription for Natural Cures: By James F. Balch M.D, Mark Stengler N.M.D. (Author), Robin Young Balch N.D. (Contributor) 2016

Natural Remedies: Natural Remedies that Heal, Protect and Provide Instant Relief from Everyday Common Ailments, Kasia Roberts, 2004

The End of Diabetes: The Eat to Live Plan to Prevent and Reverse Diabetes. HarperCollins Publications, 2014

CPSIA information can be obtained
at www.ICGtesting.com
Printed in the USA
BVHW052210281221
625055BV00008B/647